INTERDISCIPLINARY EXPANSIONS IN ENGINEERING AND DESIGN WITH THE POWER OF BIOMIMICRY

Edited by **Gulden Kokturk**
and **Tutku Didem Akyol Altun**

Interdisciplinary Expansions in Engineering and Design With the Power of Biomimicry
http://dx.doi.org/10.5772/65987
Edited by Gulden Kokturk and Tutku Didem Akyol Altun

Contributors

Ayça Tokuç, Feyzal Ozkaban, Özge Andiç Çakır, Julien R Serres, Thierry Darmanin, Sabri Taleb, Frédéric Guittard, Petra Gruber, Tim McGinley, Manuel Muehlbauer, Irem Deniz, Tugba Keskin, Maria Lorena Lehman, Hyunsoo Lee, Nayeon Kim

Published by InTech
Janeza Trdine 9, 51000 Rijeka, Croatia

Publishing Process Manager Romina Skomersic
Technical Editor SPi Global
Cover InTech Design team

First published March, 2018
Printed in Croatia
Legal deposit, Croatia: National and University Library in Zagreb

Additional hard copies can be obtained from orders@intechopen.com

Interdisciplinary Expansions in Engineering and Design With the Power of Biomimicry, Edited by Gulden Kokturk and Tutku Didem Akyol Altun
p. cm.
Print ISBN 978-953-51-3935-5
Online ISBN 978-953-51-3936-2

For EU product safety concerns:
IN TECH d.o.o., Prolaz Marije Krucifikse Kozulić 3, 51000 Rijeka, Croatia,
info@intechopen.com or visit our website at intechopen.com.

Meet the editors

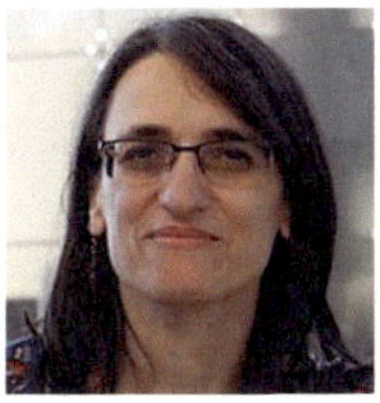

Assist. Prof. Dr. Gülden Köktürk is an electrical and electronic engineer in Dokuz Eylül University, Department of Electrical and Electronic Engineering in Izmir (Turkey). She has been working as a lecturer in Dokuz Eylül University since finishing her PhD degree. She obtained her graduate degree and PhD degree in Electrical and Electronic Engineering in 1987 and 1999, respectively. Her research interests are signal and image processing, biomedical image processing, sustainability in energy, biodesign, and biomimicry. Dr. Köktürk has published many scientific papers, conference presentations, and exhibitions. She is one of the founding members of the Turkish Biodesign Team (TBT), which is the first biodesign team of Turkey and has an interdisciplinary structure study between biomimetic, engineering, science, and design intersection. She continues to work on biodesign in science and engineering with her teammates.
Other InTech publications
Book chapter Wavelet Based Speech Strategy in Cochlear Implant by Gulden Köktürk in the book *Cochlear Implant Research Updates* edited by Cila Umat and Rinze Anthony Tange, ISBN 978-953-51-0582-4, InTech, April 4, 2012.

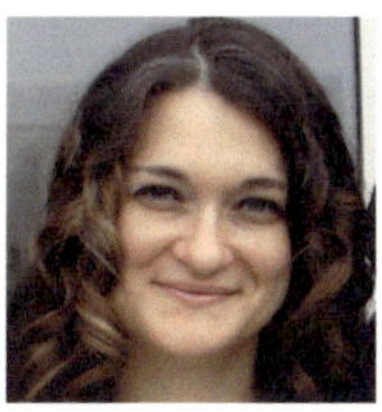

Assoc. Prof. Dr. Didem Akyol Altun is an architect in Dokuz Eylül University, Department of Architecture. She lives in Izmir (Turkey), a city located in the west of the country. She has been working at the Dokuz Eylül University as an instructor for 17 years now. She obtained her graduate degree in 2000 and PhD degree in Architecture in 2010. She deals with all areas of design and continues to work in the biomimetics, nature-inspired architecture, and design-engineering interface. She has many published scientific papers, conference presentations, exhibitions, awards from architectural competitions, and one TUBITAK (Scientific and Technological Research Council of Turkey) project coordinatorship. She is one of the founding members of the Turkish Biodesign Team (TBT), which is the first biodesign team of Turkey and has an interdisciplinary structure study between biomimetic, science, and design intersection. She continues to work on biodesign with her teammates.

Contents

Preface

Biomimicry or the similar word biomimetic comes from the unification of the Greek words "bios" (life) and "mimesis" (mimic). It was first used by the American engineer Otto Schmidt in the 1950s. Biomimicry could simply be defined as being inspired from biological forms, functions, systems, components, or processes in nature. It is also a design principle that searches for results for solving problems of humankind through analyzing nature. In contemporary approaches, biomimicry searches for a balance between nature and people. Accordingly, it suggests thinking and acting like nature instead of having a metaphorical attitude.

Biomimicry is an interdisciplinary topic related to electronics, communication, medicine, biology, chemistry, physics, math, art, and many other areas. Janine Benyus, in her book *Biomimicry: Innovation Inspired by Nature*, published in 1997, remarked on the necessity of interdisciplinary cooperation between biological research and industrial and/or construction technologies.

Biomimicry is commonly used in the design of artificial devices, prostheses, medical equipment, and robots. It is a method that has been significant in the fields of medicine, architecture, and civil engineering for many years.

The relationship between biology and design is based first on biomimicry. The process can be summarized as inspiring/adapting/learning from nature. This interaction seems to have had different forms over the years and is called biomorphic, metaphoric, or analogic approaches in the design literature. However, implied samples are completely formal inspirations, revealed from natural organisms. This attitude of mimesis was transformed at the end of the twentieth century with the notion of biomimesis and biodesign. The design practice of this period contains a conscious learning and inference goal from nature in terms of materials, structural generation, and systematic process rather than formal analogies. The target is to design products that really work as part of nature. We can call this new approach biodesign.

The investigation of living organisms at the molecular scale opens up probable ways to inspire from the genetics of organisms. Even using living organisms in design can be used as an example. Designers use different data from many science areas such as architecture, design, biotechnology, nanotechnology, biology, math, geometry, physics, chemistry, etc. Accordingly, interdisciplinary relationships between different fields are inevitable in the twenty-first century.

Biomimicry has now brought together engineers and designers, and this collaboration creates innovative and creative outcomes. Nevertheless, more research is needed in this area because many studies on biomimicry are generally about the health sector. It can be said that engineering studies come in second place. However, there are a few studies on design and biomimicry from an interdisciplinary point of view. Similarly, interdisciplinary foundations between science, engineering, and design are very few globally. Undoubtedly, there are a number of strong foundations or teams in Europe, America, and East Asia. But their concern is biodesign in medical science. So new studies, both foundational and theoretical in between design, science, and engineering, are clearly a necessity. Accordingly, this book aims to fill this gap in the literature.

The book contains eight chapters from expert and well-known authors in their fields. Petra Gruber, Tim McGinley, and Manuel Muehlbauer in their chapter "Towards an Agile Biodigital Architecture: Supporting a Dynamic Evolutionary and Developmental View of Architecture" are focused on a strategic methodology for architectural design processes using evolutionary and genetic principles. They used the potential of computer science that links biological concept to architectural application by making a bridge between biology and design. The authors actualized five parallel workshops to explore their biological concept in design and tried to generate an active design tool based on agile principles integrating biological models in a new multistage design process. The inputs of their work are a dynamic representation of the explored typology of the South Australian House.

Maria Lorena Lehman deals with designing an optimization method for communication between buildings by using a biomimetic approach to derive lessons from the human eye and its focusing abilities. She suggests this method to uplift the urban quality of life by transforming the buildings—which are often static without adapting to the ever-changing context that surrounds them—into "communication bridges" in her chapter "Human Eye Behaviors Inform Systems Design for Inter-Building Communication."

Inspired robot design by nature is widely used. By considering this point, Julien Serres tries to bring a different perspective to drone miniaturization and navigation inside buildings. In his chapter "Taking Inspiration from Flying Insects to Navigate Inside Buildings," bio-inspired sensors and optic flow-based direct feedback loops were applied to a micro air vehicle and this design has been demonstrated for a drone flying inside buildings.

Regarding the relationship between biology and design, we could mention "bio-cooperation" as a new approach in the twenty-first century. It is noticed that using living organisms and nature in design is beyond inspiring . In this context, the next two chapters are concerned with hybrid design synthesis between biology and design collaboration.

İrem Deniz and Tuğba Keskin Gündoğdu introduce the use of living organisms in the design area from a bioengineer's point of view. The possible uses of bacteria, microalgae, and fungi in biomimetic design are briefly discussed in their chapter "Biomimetic Design for a Bioengineered World." They also mention biomaterials for biodesign. Using the potential of bacteria, fungi, and microalgal strains in the building creates an exciting balance between cost-effective, non-toxic, and natural characteristics. The authors also noticed that interdisciplinary cooperation could be utilized to develop bio-based products in the future.

In the chapter "Biomimetic Façade Applications for a More Sustainable Future," Ayça Tokuç, F. Feyzal Özkaban, and Özge Andiç Çakır look at the possibilities of biomimetics and biodesign methods in sustainable façade designs. They introduce the design principles of sustainable façades first, and then related construction materials and some contemporary examples are explained. The authors mention the harmony between the concept of biomimicry and sustainability but point out that every biomimetic application is not always sustainable. They suggest bio-cooperation with natural elements in façade design as another way to learn from nature.

These two chapters also mention a biodesign team in Turkey, Turkey Biodesign Team, that is promising for Eastern European countries.

Hyunsoo Lee and Nayeon Kim in a chapter called "Bio-inspired Adaptable Façade Control Reflecting User's Behavior" present the process of methodology for designing an adaptable façade to change environments and requirements for humans. The design of the adaptable façade inspired from nature is also one of the main reasons for the work to be included in this book. Moreover, biomimetic façade control is implemented in the content.

In nature, many plants and animals have superhydrophobic properties. These superhydrophic properties provide us with new technological products by focusing on these living beings. In the chapter "Switchable and Reversible Superhydrophobic Surfaces," parts one and two, written by Sabri Taleb, Thierry Darmanin, and Frédéric Guittard, a superhydrophobic surface is described. Surfaces with robust superhydrophobic properties are needed for practical applications. This work presents how a superhydrophobic surface is able to be stabilized in the Cassie-Baxter state.

Reading and interpreting the chapters of this book as editors, we have learned many things during the process. We are very appreciative to all contributing authors for their efforts and to dear Romina Skomersic, our publishing process manager, and Anja Filipovic, our commissioning editor, for their patience and endeavor.

It would appear that the twenty-first century is producing many new and amazing designs. Before these educative and exciting processes can be combined, this book will be an important guide to take a quick look at all the possibilities.

Gulden Kokturk
Dokuz Eylül University, Turkey

Tutku Didem Akyol Altun
Dokuz Eylül niversity, Turkey

Chapter 1

Towards an Agile Biodigital Architecture: Supporting a Dynamic Evolutionary and Developmental View of Architecture

Petra Gruber, Tim McGinley and
Manuel Muehlbauer

Additional information is available at the end of the chapter

http://dx.doi.org/10.5772/intechopen.72916

Abstract

Architecture and biology are fields of high complexity. Generative design approaches provide access to continuously increasing complexity in design. Some of these methods are based on biological principles but usually do not communicate the conceptual base necessary to appropriately reflect the input from biology into architecture. To address this, we propose a model for analysis and design of architecture based on a multistaged integrated design process that extends the common morphological process in digital morphogenesis with a typology-based ontological model. Biomimetics, an emerging field to strategically search for information transfer from biology to technological application, will assist in delivering a frame of reference and methodology for establishing valid analogies between the different realms as well as integration of the biological concept into a larger framework of analogy to biological processes. As the biomimetic translation of process and systems information promises more radical innovation, this chapter focuses on the dynamic perspectives provided by biological development and evolution to model the complexity of architecture. The proposed process was used to inform five parallel workshops to explore dynamic biological concepts in design. The potential of the process to investigate biomimetic processes in architecture is then discussed, and future work is outlined.

Keywords: biomimetics, evolutionary design, morphogenesis, morphogenetic prototyping, agile design principles

1. Introduction

This chapter identifies a multistaged integrated design process for the analysis and design of architecture, which extends the common morphological process with a typology-based ontological model. Architecture involves the design, control and manipulation of a multitude of complex systems to result in a successful building. Therefore, there is a continuous exploration of the transfer of models from external disciplines into architecture to support modelling and ultimately the control of this complexity. For instance, generative design allows the exploration of various design solutions based on the definition of design-specific representations and generative rules and behaviours, which allow to iteratively generate designs in a bottom-up process.

Some of these methods are based on biological principles [1–3], and as evolutionary theories in biology are radically revised [4, 5], the terminology in this context needs to be revisited to include novel biological concepts. Biomimetics provides methods to communicate the conceptual base from biology into design and has promoted novel approaches to architectural design [6]. Morphological processes targeting formfinding have previously been explored in digital morphogenesis [7–9]. Additionally, McGinley [10] proposed a framework to support the integration of concepts of biological development into architectural design while also exploring the concept of agile design. Therefore, we propose and discuss a method to support designers to integrate biological concepts of development and evolution in their work.

At the same time, it is important to caution that biology is a broad discipline, which is built from a multitude of perspectives. Tinbergen defined these as the four questions of biology. The questions divide biology into dynamic and static views which are then each subdivided into how and why questions. The dynamic views consider why the organism evolved and how it developed into the biological artefact, whereas the static view interrogates a biological artefact at a single point in time. In biomimetics, this is paralleled by material, structural, process or systems translations from nature into technology.

Computer science links biological concepts to architectural application, serving as a bridge between biology and design. Therefore, this chapter applies adapted agile design methods from computer science in architecture, proposing a strategy for translation of biological observation on a system level to computational design systems in architecture using evolutionary and genetic principles. To create a test bed for this conceptual approach, a design workshop event 'Agile X4' focusing on the South Australian housing typologies was organised to create a proof of concept case study.

2. Evolution in design

Evolution and natural selection are characteristic signs of life, which result in a continuous improvement of the biosphere by providing resilience, adaptation and development. These properties are also desired in architectural design processes. Therefore, a review of the evolutionary concepts in the realm of architecture seems to be a promising approach to build on the recent developments in evolutionary architecture that adopt a computer science method for the generative development of design solutions. Evolution as a strategy has been applied to a technical context as an optimization strategy since Ingo Rechenberg pioneered evolutionary computation in the 1970s [11, 12]. Rechenberg's Evolutionary Strategy (ES) served to solve complex optimization questions in science that could not yet be tackled by theoretical approaches. This methodology is aimed at improving technical optimization and is thus embedded in the context of technology.

The architectural discourse about the use of evolutionary computation in generative design processes is based on the introduction of Genetic Algorithms, developed by Holland [13] and Genetic Programming, introduced by Koza [14] to the scripting practice for architectural design tools. The pioneering work of Frazer [1] provides a strong knowledge base for architectural designers to come to explore the possible applications of evolutionary computation. In the section on genetic language, Frazer points out that multiple levels of representations determine the genetic hierarchy required to develop a living organism. Additionally, there is potential for the use of language characteristic elements, vocabulary and syntax, as described by Contreras and Chomsky [15–17]. In this context, the complexity of representation for architectural design is already tangible.

Recent developments in computer science that use grammatical evolution [18–20] extend the repertoire of generative design strategies with an evolutionary approach using a reduced representation even for complex design cases. These systems build on the rule-based approach in shape grammar [21], but encompass the potential to drive the unfolding of computational designs based on behavioural systems in bottom-up processes.

3. Biomimetics

Biomimetics, an emerging field to strategically search for information transfer from biology to technological application, assists in delivering a generic frame of reference and methodology for establishing valid analogies between different realms. Defined as an innovation methodology, the process of biomimetics involves basic research, abstraction of principles and translation of those principles into an application field. Biomimetics deals with materials, structures and systems, but typically extracts knowledge about functions, mechanism or concepts that are then applied by designers or interpreted by engineers. Moreover, the interdisciplinarity inherent in biomimetics holds the potential for radical, new innovations and sustainable products and technologies [22].

Biomimetics has been increasingly explored in the context of architecture, design and the arts in the last decade, and a biological paradigm seems to underlie current trends in design research [23]. Examples for biomimetic applications at the scale of materials and surfaces are self-cleaning or easy-to-clean coatings on glass and metals and also facade paint. Structures and constructions informed from biology, especially from plant structures, are explored in prototypical buildings like the ICD/ITKE pavilions and also include products like flectofin, a novel facade-shading system using a compliant mechanism inspired by the opening mechanism of the flower of the bird-of-paradise (*Strelitzia reginae*) [6]. Most recently, aliveness of architecture is discussed within the context of growth of material structures and agency. Growth principles from biology are increasingly explored in computation, generating a new morphological space that is transferred into material systems by additive production technologies like 3D printing. Metabolic activity as a base for all life is also explored in architectural design by creating matter and energy flows in prototype installations, in addition to the use of algae and bacterial as integral and active elements into wall, facade and soil systems [6, 24, 25].

Methodologies and tools for biomimetics are being developed primarily to facilitate the knowledge transfer for the technology side. Translation tools, databases such as AskNature [26] and methodologies such as BioTriz [27] have not been introduced on a large scale yet. A very concise description of the process of biomimetics can be found in the German VDI Standard [22] and in publications of the Biologically Inspired Design at the Georgia Tech Institute [12]. A new and intriguing way forward is the development of an ontology for biomimetics [28]. Ontologies deal with the definition of entities and their relations. Biological principles can be expressed in computational representations and ontologies to inform computational design processes.

The introduction of biomimetics in the field of evolutionary and agile design allows the integration of those concepts into a larger framework of design and analogy to biological processes. It provides a methodology for analogy building, abstraction and information transfer and promotes process and systems translation into technology. As a frame concept, biomimetics requires a reinterpretation of mimicking evolutionary processes in design. Apart from material representations of architecture referring to biological materials and structures, phylogenetic history and genetics of the role model refer to dynamic translations and distinctive design processes.

4. Agile design

Project management methods can be defined as either predictive or adaptive. Predictive models rely on the information of the project being fixed at the start of the project and that which is unknown being accurately predicted. Alternatively, adaptive methods support variability in the requirements and constraints of a project. Samset and Volden [29] propose a series of paradoxes of predictive project management. These can be summarised in that many important decisions about a design project need to be made at its start, when we know the least about the project. The strategic errors resulting from these myopic decisions are further frustrated by any misalignment of the selected tactical approach to realise the chosen strategy.

Alternatively, the founders of the agile movement defined a manifesto [30] with a set of principles for supporting a more adaptive approach to the development of software. The fourth principle, responding to change over following a plan, provides the underlying principle for agile design. Agile design approaches achieve this by working in cycles so that decision making can be more flexible (agile) and changes can be made later. Built environment projects are traditionally predictive, which can mean that changes can be difficult to implement. One major advantage of biomimetics is that it provides a broad body of potential solutions for a project but that implementation of each example requires the design model to adapt. Therefore, we propose that employing agile design principles in architecture could support further exploration of the design opportunity space which will better support the implementation of dynamic biomimetic concepts in architecture [31].

Furthermore, the model abstraction provided by the computational lens allows for a deeper investigation of the biological analogy of evolution and architecture and expands the knowledge transfer to have a direct impact on the process of architectural conceptualisation. In this way, computational design approaches such as evolutionary programming and agile design support adaption of design models of continuously increasing complexity in design.

5. Multistage design process

To support biomimetic concepts such as evolutionary design in architecture, this chapter employs agile design concepts to facilitate the exploration of the opportunity space of architectural design. This is proposed here in an abstract model for the analysis and design of architecture based on a multistage design process. This process uses the following stages of (1) identifying the features of the design; (2) extracting pseudo-genes from the features; (3) establishing the phenotype (what the evolved and developed typology would look like) and finally (4) altering the genes and repeating the previous steps. In this way, the process extends the common morphological process in digital morphogenesis with a typology-based ontological model.

5.1. Identify the features

In the first stage, the features of the typologies are identified as the input data for the system. These features could include distinct architectural elements, spatial entities and relationships that characterise the typologies. This process results in a feature matrix that can be translated into a computational system.

5.2. Define the genes

This phase identifies the 'genes' of the design, based on the feature matrix. In an analogy to reverse engineering, existing features lead back to the rules of creation. These rules could be thought of as design genes [10, 32].

5.3. Model the phenotype

The next stage is to generate virtual phenotypes based on the feature matrix and design genes. McGinley et al. [33] proposed that the architectural phenotype is based on environmental influences on the (architectural) genotype. For modelling the phenotype, there are several options:

- A model based on voxels – dividing the space up into boxes that could then be spatially allocated
- A model that we describe as a 'bag of beans', which involves a randomly distributed but static set of 'nuclei' that are grouped, shelled or hulled depending on the spatial position information

- A dynamic computational fluid dynamics model wherein the nuclei (cells or beans) can move and be moved by gradient forces inside the pseudo-organism.

5.4. Modify the phenotype

The virtual representation of the phenotype is evaluated in a selection process. Evaluation can take place against a chosen set of criteria in the digital realm, or can introduce modification by external influence in a virtual reality environment. A modified phenotype results from this phase. Feedback from this last phase can then connect back to the input data or abstracted gene stage. In order to trace the flow back to the initial data stage, a real world translation is required.

6. Case study (Agile X4: morphogenetic prototyping)

The Agile X4 event at the University of South Australia in Adelaide served as a test bed for the conceptual approach. The proposed workflow of the integrated design system requires the collaboration of multiple disciplines: architecture theory, data experts, biology, computational design, computer science and programming, virtual reality experts. The integration of multidisciplinary design teams generates the necessity for the establishment of communication protocols on both the level of human interaction and the level of systems interaction. The validity of the proposed model was investigated in the workshop event called 'Agile X4'. During the timeframe of 1 week, five parallel workshops were conducted with an international team of 29 researchers and students. Together, the five workshops covered the workflow described in the previous chapter, mapping the workshop activities to the integrated design process (**Table 1**).

The workshops started simultaneously and ran over 5 days, with an integrated conference and synthesis time to coordinate and connect the results. The activities, tools and methods of each phase are described here based on the workflow model of the multistage design process (**Figure 1**). The main flow of information was established, leading from research in architecture

Workshop	Description	Input	Define	Model	Modify
Carve	Prototype a tangible user interface (beyond pencil, keyboard and mouse) [34] for multistage process				✓
Design X	Define a VR experience for defining and altering the phenotypes			✓	✓
Evo Type	Provide an evolutionary perspective on the history of the South Australian House and identify its 'genes' and adaptations over time	✓	✓		✓
Reverse	View the typical Adelaide house as if it had developed biologically		✓		✓
BioMod	Develop the generative explicit geometry for the case study			✓	✓

Table 1. Mapping of the parallel workshops of Agile X4 to the integrated design stages.

http://dx.doi.org/10.5772/intechopen.72916

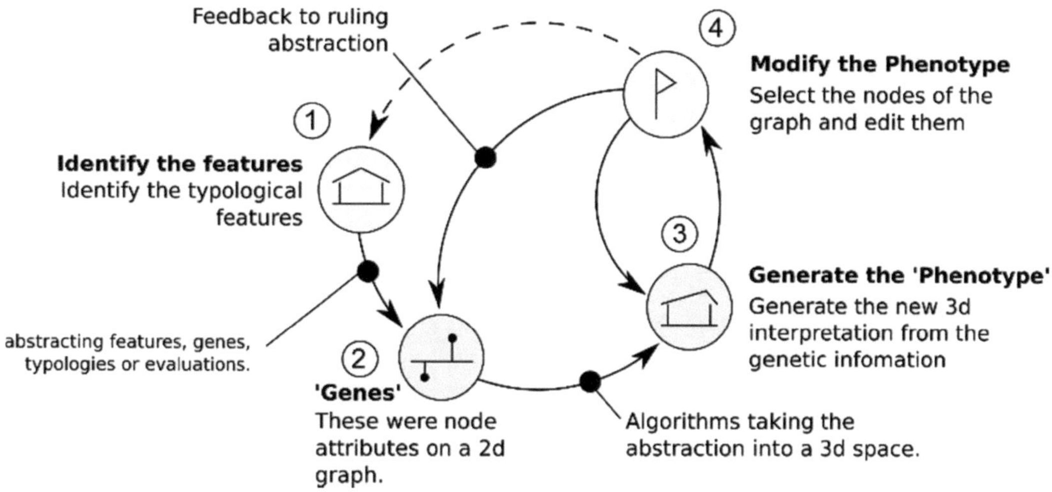

Figure 1. Stages of the agile biodigital design process.

history over typological interpretation, abstraction of spatial information into topology diagrams and ontologies, creating organismic analogies by differentiation into body plans, translation into an analogy to genetic information, generation of a new spatial interpretation based on environmental parameters and modification using interface tools in a virtual environment to finally feeding the modified information back into the cycle.

6.1. Identify the features

South Australian housing typologies were used as the base architectural input model. In collaboration with UniSA Architecture Museum, a literature research and archive research were carried out, and a set of building drawings selected and analysed. This enabled the identification and selection of specific features that were then encoded in a diagrammatic topological map and a feature matrix of the houses along with the basic data including, for example, date of construction.

6.2. Encode the genes

The next stage based on the feature matrix was to identify the 'genes' of the design. Spatial features of the South Australia houses were translated into connectivity diagrams (**Figure 2**). The Evo Type workshop provided an evolutionary perspective on the history of the South Australian House. It was then possible to model a developmental perspective for each typology based on a hierarchy derived from its connectivity diagram.

6.3. Generate the phenotype

The graphs (connectivity diagrams) generated in the gene encoding stage were sent from Grasshopper to control pheromone growth of a particle system in Maya that was rendered in real time as a series of boxes in Unity (**Figure 3**).

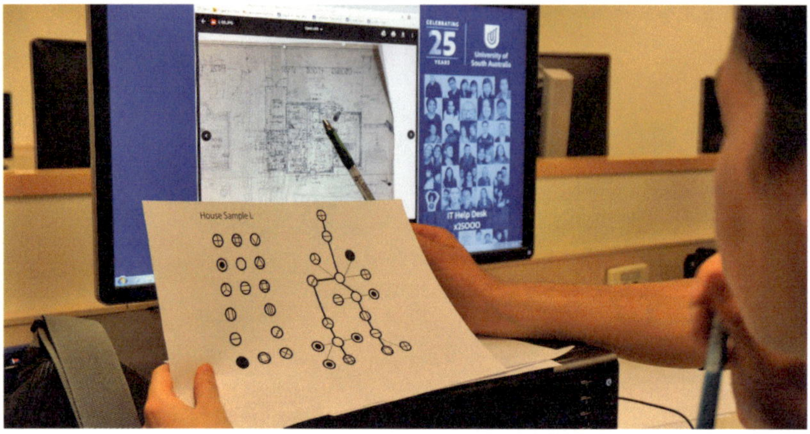

Figure 2. Adelaide house types with their connectivity graphs (photo credit, Petra Gruber).

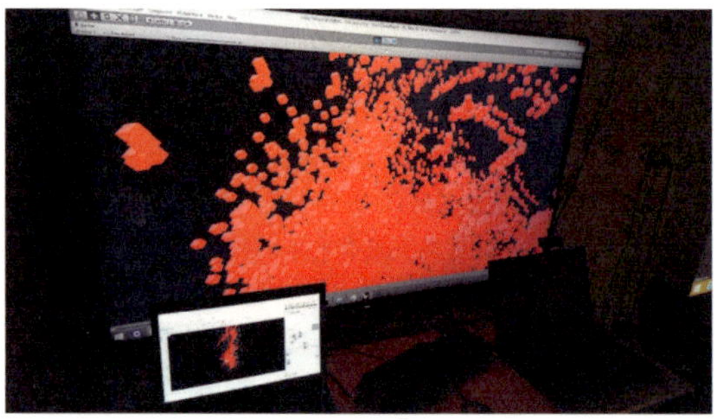

Figure 3. The generated phenotype based on the connectivity diagram interpreted in grasshopper and Maya into Unity.

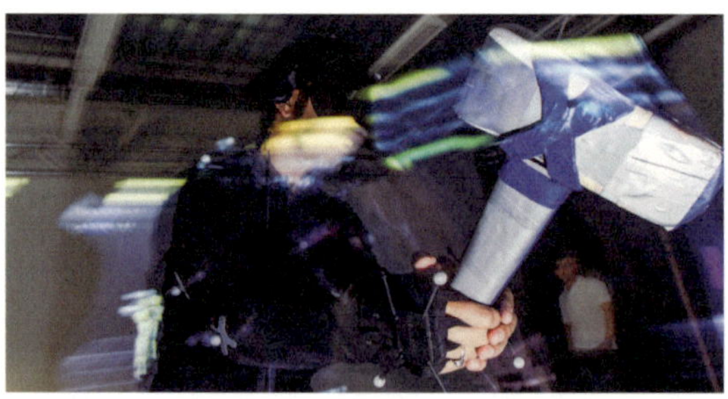

Figure 4. Design X workshop tutor Daish Malani testing the gene adaptation prototype agile 'axe' (photo credit, Kelly Carpenter).

6.4. Modify the phenotype

In parallel, the carve workshop produced a tangible user interface prototype in the form of an axe. This enabled the user to select and modify specific nodes in the connectivity diagram in a virtual reality space, thereby altering the pseudo-body plan of the architectural typology (**Figure 4**).

7. Results and discussion

During the translation of knowledge from developmental biology to architectural design, we realised the immense potential to extend morphogenetic design methodologies. In response to the changing perspective on evolutionary and developmental processes in biology, the architectural interpretation of morphogenetic design was revisited. The extension of the evolutionary design model with a typological ontogeny was facilitated in an iterative design process. During the process, the knowledge about the problem was built in multiple groups, each responsible for a stage in the explored multistaged design model. After an advanced design state was achieved in one of the groups, the integration with neighbouring groups in the design model led to an increased level of integration. At this crucial moment, knowledge was successively transferred between interacting groups to provide an embedded understanding of the process. As a result, a rigorous argument was developed to communicate between groups. Evidence of the design process inside the distinct groups was used to transfer and communicate embodied knowledge between those groups. The research on a new multistage design process provided a validation of the comparison of genetics and architectural typology and an extension of the basic analogy of evolutionary architecture.

The agile process of the workshop allowed us to develop the communication model for the integrated design system on the fly. The communication protocol and initial workflow of the design system were developed, implemented and tested during the workshops. Limitations and challenges were found in the translation between the distinct phases. Building a shared computational representation during the workshop was the biggest challenge. The initial desire to translate implicit knowledge stored in traditional typologies to modern design approaches was not fully reached based on the time constraints. A prototypical software implementation for a design process that would be able to facilitate reaching this goal was investigated and tested. The outcome of the workshop was therefore a result of a rigorous investigation on the geometric translation and computational communication of the implicit knowledge inside the explored topology. As a result, an interactive methodology for a multistaged adaptive design system was successfully tested using an abstract geometrical representation. The selection mechanism in a virtual environment was crucial to the overall success. Here, the concept was the manipulation of the graph model based on the user input. As this was not tested in a closed-loop system before, the potential of the user guidance of the design process through gesture has yet to be explored. The main barrier to implementation during the workshop was the complexity of the data that should be mapped from the gesture to the computational model. Overall, the use of a persistent graph model for the testing of computational design systems proved to be a feasible approach to reduce the system complexity. It allowed to test the workflow in the brief period of the workshops.

8. Conclusion

This chapter proposes the development of a system to design active tools based on agile principles integrating biological models in a new multi-stage design process. The combination of an agile approach on the level of human interaction with the use of biomimetic principles on the systems level allowed us to establish efficient protocols and use the synergetic effects between computational design systems in architecture and systems design based on biomimetic principles. The multistage computational model was developed and tested in an initial design experiment of Agile X4.

The outcome of the workshop series was in many respects promising:

- The results of the feature matrix during the definition of the ontological input were successfully used to generate a dynamic representation of the explored typology of the South Australian House.
- The main advantage of the agile approach is the modularity of the system that is based on the specification of a communication protocol shared over all stages of the design process. It allowed the use of a variety of design tools that are available in the CAD software packages of Rhinoceros, Maya and Unity. A developmental model for generative design was used to develop a flexible graph model as communication protocol in the computational design system.
- Based on the developed design system, further investigations on geometrically refined representations promise to transfer additional knowledge from the traditional typology to state-of-the-art computational design processes capable of exploring large design spaces.

There is an enormous potential for form generation in reference to existing typologies using the developed multistage design system. Furthermore, a four-dimensional mapping of the genotypes to the phenotypes would encourage speculation about topological changes introduced by the aliveness of architecture.

9. Future work

The further development of the proposed multistage design process entails improvements on various levels. Firstly, the basic analogy between architectural design and evolutionary development should be revisited and recent findings in the life sciences integrated into the translation. Novel concepts such as niche construction theory and epigenetics have not been sufficiently discussed in the context of the built environment.

Secondly, for the distinct phases of the design process, further research would provide further understanding of the flexibility inherent in the design system. So, for the gene extraction, the number of features that are mapped between genotype and phenotype should be increased, and for the phenotype modelling, the mapping of building features in a particle system would drive the development of the phenotype through existing typologies. The implementation of a flexible graph model would allow the mapping of the defined genotype on a four-dimensional space-time model. Additional research should also be conducted on the behaviour of the system interaction of different typologies with each other (ecology simulation). The relation of typologies to environmental context is another interesting field of research that could be further investigated in a comparative study over different climatic and cultural zones.

Acknowledgements

The research presented here was supported by UniSA's Research Theme Investment Scheme Seed funding. The Agile X4 workshops promoted a flat hierarchy between tutors and participants who included the authors in alphabetical order: Alex Degaris-Boot, Andrew Lymm-Penning, Aurélien Forget, Brett Abroe, Claire Timpani, Conor Mannering, Daish Malani, Daniela Mitterberger, Fraser Murison, Gwilyn Saunders, James Wilson, Julie Collins, Kei Hoshi, Kelly Carpenter, Linus Tan, Mark Langman, Nimish Biloria, Patrick Scott, Roxane Adams, Shane Haddy, Simon Biggs, Thomas Kuys, Gwilyn Saunders, Timothy Tuppence, Tiziano Derme and William Mount.

Author details

Petra Gruber[1]*, Tim McGinley[2] and Manuel Muehlbauer[3]

*Address all correspondence to: pgruber@uakron.edu

1 University of Akron, Biomimicry Research and Innovation Center, Akron, USA

2 University of South Australia, Adelaide, Australia

3 RMIT, Melbourne, Australia

References

[1] Frazer J. An Evolutionary Architecture. London: Architectural Association; 1995 (Themes, 7)

[2] Janssen P. A Design Method and Computational Architecture for Generating and Evolving Building Designs. Dissertation. Hong Kong: The Hong Kong Polytechnic University, School of Design; 2005

[3] Fernando R. Representations for Evolutionary Design Modelling. Dissertation. Queensland: Queensland University of Technology, School of Design; 2014

[4] Noble D. Evolution beyond neo-Darwinism: A new conceptual framework. The Journal of Experimental Biology. 2015;**218**(Pt 1):7-13. DOI: 10.1242/jeb.106310

[5] Laland KN, Uller T, Feldman MW, Sterelny K, Muller GB, Moczek A, et al. The extended evolutionary synthesis: Its structure, assumptions and predictions. Proceedings of Biological sciences. 2015;**282**(1813):20151019. DOI: 10.1098/rspb.2015.1019

[6] Knippers J, Nickel KG, Speck T. Biomimetic Research for Architecture and Building Construction. Switzerland: Springer International Publishing; 2016

[7] Roudavski A. Towards morphogenesis in architecture. International Journal of Architectural Computing. 2009;**7**(3):345-374. DOI: 10.1260/147807709789621266

[8] Menges A. Computational morphogenesis: Integral form generation and materialization processes. In: Okeil A, Al-Attili A, Mallasi Z, editors. Proceedings of Em'body'ing

Virtual Architecture: The Third International Conference of the Arab Society for Computer Aided Architectural Design ASCAAD 2007, Alexandria, Egypt. Nov 28-30, 2007. pp. 725-744

[9] Hensel M, Menges A, Weinstock M. Techniques and technologies in morphogenetic design. In: Architectural Design. Vol. 76(2). London: Wiley-Academy; 2006. Available from: http://onlinelibrary.wiley.com/1850-9999

[10] McGinley T. A morphogenetic architecture for intelligent buildings. Intelligent Buildings International. Nov. 2015;**7**(1):4-15

[11] Rechenberg I. Evolutionsstrategie – Optimierung technischer Systeme nach Prinzipien der biologischen Evolution [PhD thesis]. TU Berlin, Germany, 1971

[12] Goel A, McAdams DA, Stone RB. Biologically Inspired Design—Computational Methods and Tools. London, UK: Springer; 2014

[13] Holland J. Genetic algorithms and the optimal allocation of trials. SIAM Journal on Computing. 1973;**2**(2):88-105. DOI: 10.1137/0202009

[14] Koza JR. Genetic Programming. A Paradigm for Genetically Breeding Populations of Computer Programs to Solve Problems. Stanford, CA: Stanford University. Department of Computer Science; 1990

[15] Contreras H, Chomsky N. Aspects of the theory of syntax. The Modern Language Journal. 1967;**51**(2):1-10. DOI: 10.2307/321826

[16] Chomsky N. Syntactic Structures. The Hague/Paris: Mouton; 1975. ISBN: 978-3-11-021832-9

[17] Chomsky N. Rules and Representations. Oxford: Blackwell; 1980

[18] Muehlbauer M, Song A, Burry J. Automated shape design by grammatical evolution. Vol. 10198. In: Correia J, Ciesielski V, Liapis A, editors. Computational Intelligence in Music, Sound, Art and Design. 6th International Conference on EvoMUSART 2017, Amsterdam, The Netherlands, April 19-21, 2017. LNCS Sublibrary SL 1, Theoretical Computer Science and General Issues. Cham, Switzerland: Springer; 2017. Available online at http://link.springer.com/

[19] O'Neill M, McDermott J, Swafford JM, Byrne J, Hemberg E, Brabazon A, et al. Evolutionary design using grammatical evolution and shape grammars. Designing a shelter. International Journal of Difference Equations. 2010;**3**(1):4. DOI: 10.1504/IJDE.2010.032820

[20] Byrne J. Approaches to Evolutionary Architectural Design Exploration Using Grammatical Evolution. Dissertation. Dublin: University College Dublin; 2012

[21] Stiny G, Gips J. Shape grammars and the generative specification of painting and sculpture. In: Information Processing. Vol. 71. Amsterdam: North-Holland Publishing Company; 1972. pp. 1460-1465

[22] VDI (Verein Deutscher Ingenieure) Guideline 6220. Biomimetics – Conception and strategy differences between bionic and conventional methods/products. Association of German Engineers. Berlin: Beuth Verlag; 2011

[23] Gruber P. Biomimetics in Architecture—Architecture of Life and Buildings. Wien, Austria: Springer; 2011

[24] Imhof B, Gruber P, editors. Built to Grow: Blending Architecture and Biology. Birkhäuser, Basel, Switzerland: Edition Angewandte; 2015

[25] Armstrong R. Vibrant Architecture: Matter as a CoDesigner of Living Structures. Warsaw/Berlin: de Gruyter; 2015

[26] Deldin JM, Schuknecht M. The AskNature database: Enabling solutions in biomimetic design. In: Goel A, McAdams D, Stone R, editors. Biologically Inspired Design. London: Springer; 2014; pp. 17-27

[27] Bogatyrev N, Bogatyreva O. BioTRIZ: A win-win methodology for eco-innovation. Vol. 2. In: Azevedo S, Brandenburg M, Carvalho H, Cruz-Machado V, editors. Eco-Innovation and the Development of Business Models. Greening of Industry Networks Studies. Cham: Springer; 2014; pp. 297-314

[28] Vincent J. An ontology of Biomimetics. In: Goel AK, McAdams DA, Stone RB, editors. Biologically Inspired Design, Computational Methods and Tools. London, UK: Springer; 2014. pp. 269-285

[29] Samset K, Volden GH. Front-end definition of projects: Ten paradoxes and some reflections regarding project management and project governance. International Journal of Project Management. 2016;**34**(2):297-313

[30] Beck K, Beedle M, van Bennekum A, Cockburn A, Cunningham W, Fowler M, Grenning J, Highsmith J, Hunt A, Jeffries R, Kern J, Marick B, Martin RC, Mellor S, Schwaber K, Sutherland J, Thomas D. Manifesto for Agile Software Development. 2001. Available from: http://agilemanifesto.org/ [2017-04]

[31] McGinley T, Abroe B, Kroll D, Sare T, Gu N: Agile X Pavilion: Agile principles and the parametric paradox. 22nd Annual Conference of the Association for Computer-Aided Architectural Design Research in Asia, Suzhou, China; 2017

[32] Gero JS, Kazakov VA. Evolving design genes in space layout planning problems. Artificial Intelligence in Engineering. 1998;**12**:163-176

[33] McGinley T, Collins J, Schwarz Q, Muehlbauer M. Suburban Mutations: Towards the Multi-Dimensional Appropriation of Science in Architecture. Architectural Science Association; 2016

[34] McGinley T, Hoshi K, Iacopetta L. MorphoCarve: Carving morphogenetic prototypes. 6th Conference of the International Association of Societies of Design Research, Brisbane, Australia; 2015

Chapter 2

Human Eye Behaviors Inform Systems Design for Inter-Building Communication

Maria Lorena Lehman

Additional information is available at the end of the chapter

http://dx.doi.org/10.5772/intechopen.72911

Abstract

Adaptive sensory environments optimize in real time to consistently improve performance. One optimization method involves communication between buildings to dramatically compound positive effects—but the way these buildings communicate, matters. To design such a communication framework, this chapter uses a biomimetic approach to derive lessons from the human eye and its focusing abilities. With each focusing action, coordination occurs as muscles move to expand and contract the eye's lens to achieve varying focal distances. And when both eyes focus together, they are able to achieve stereopsis, a field of depth and perception not attainable with only the focus of one eye. By dissecting this collaboration between eye muscle coordination and stereopsis, this chapter uncovers how a communication framework between adaptive sensory environments can create indirect, yet powerful, collective occupant and building behaviors. For example, communicating adaptive sensory environments evoke greener occupant behaviors, which, in turn, bring added benefit to the natural environment. Communication framework aspects include gamification, social media, and augmented reality that blur the boundaries between built-environments in different ways. These "communication bridges" allow buildings to take on new symbiotic relationships with each other to harness and enhance how entire urban areas uplift quality of life.

Keywords: adaptive architecture, interactive architecture, sensory design, biomimicry, eye accommodation, inter-building communication, green design, occupant-centered design

1. Introduction

Buildings within urban areas today already communicate to a certain extent. Communication is inherent within their design, as a building's architect must create an environment that "speaks" to its surrounding context of other buildings through its design. In other words, as a design is being realized, it is responding to its future surrounding context as its architect imagines it into being. Yet, once constructed, the design is often static, as it stands without adapting to the ever-changing context that surrounds it.

At times, such buildings work hard to meet certain needs and goals, but because they do not adapt to changing demands and desires, they remain limited. Also, there are times where other buildings within an urban area may conflict with the way a particular building reaches certain individual or collective goals. In this case, another building can actually undo the hard work a different particular building has been designed to do.

Thus, the way buildings communicate today is often fragmented, contradictory, and static. This is why it is important to better understand how buildings can use communication in positive ways that strengthen their design and performance. By thinking and designing consciously about the inter-building communication network within an urban area, new goals can be achieved in dynamic ways. After all, communication between architecture is more than just about making a statement; it becomes more about designing for consistent optimization for learning—where a design, once built, improves over time as it communicates.

This chapter serves as a guide on how to design a framework for inter-building communication by taking a biomimetic approach that parallels eye accommodation (eye focusing) and stereopsis in vision to how buildings can communicate to focus and harness performance. In simplest terms, the human eyes work together as a team that serves as a model for how to design inter-communicating buildings. This framework allows building communication to advance greatly as it would no longer be fragmented, contradictory, and static. Instead, communication between buildings would be convergent, collaborative, and adaptive.

For buildings to communicate successfully, they must pull from the power of adaptive sensory environments. These buildings are prime for an urban communication network since they are sensory designed environments that engage with occupants, other buildings, and surrounding contexts, in dynamic and adaptive ways. For this reason, inter-building communication for adaptive sensory environments holds the most promise for positive benefit at city-wide and individual levels.

This chapter demonstrates why such inter-building communication is important, as well as illustrating how, by learning from the design of the human eyes, it can be designed to work for maximum value at all scales.

2. Adaptive sensory environments improve performance

Built-environments are gaining in their ability to not only interact with occupants and their surrounding context, but to also adapt. This occurs as new developments in sensor technology become integrated along with emerging design processes. Together, they yield environments that change in real time to meet occupant short-term needs and longer-term goals [1].

Within adaptive sensory environments, static and transient materials work together tuning to occupants, supporting them both directly and indirectly. This stems from the occupant-centered approach to design, which holds sensory design as a guiding principle. By adjusting a building's characteristics moment-by-moment, it becomes possible to not only meet a one-time occupant need but also meet ongoing occupant needs, which help achieve longer-term goals through processes such as learning.

Adaptive sensory environments bring great benefit to occupants because they allow for greater personalization through real-time tuning. This creates built-environments that do not just "house" function, but proactively work to "foster" function. For example, this is the difference between a hospital that contains healing, versus a hospital that nurtures healing [1]. In other words, the hospital environment becomes a participant of the "healing team."

In order for such adaptive buildings to function optimally, they engage in a two-way dialog with occupants. Thus, as occupants' needs and goals change and grow, the architectural environment does so as well. Each teaches and learns from the other.

In efforts to optimize such adaptive sensory environments, it is necessary to understand how communication between such buildings affects both the occupants that inhabit them as well as their surrounding natural environment. In this sense, adaptive buildings act as a "bridge" between occupants and their natural surrounding context. To do this, it is advantageous for such buildings to communicate with one another.

3. Inter-building communication for optimization

An inter-building communication network can work to help such adaptive environments cooperate and collaborate with each other. By pulling from the best of what each building does, regardless of the building type, other buildings can learn and use what works to help both their occupants and their natural surroundings. And this can all happen in real time, moment-by-moment.

When adaptive sensory environments communicate with one another, they are able to grasp a "bigger picture" of not only what their occupant needs, but also of how they can help their occupants. Thus, the boundary of a particular building may shift as its occupant and their needs shift as well. For example, a hospital may learn from its patient's home environment about how their hospital room should function regarding light levels, daily habits, or ideal temperatures within which this particular occupant can thrive.

Inter-building communication between adaptive sensory environments helps occupants both individually and collectively. Yes, the adaptive architecture tunes to a specific occupant's needs and goals, but it also can coordinate and pull from the collective needs and goals of a group, city, or culture. This allows for a type of "teamwork" to occur where the built-environment works as a conductor, helping to pull the best from occupants, while also coordinating their efforts to meet a greater good that benefits all. Thus, inter-building communication allows occupants that are located in different places at different times to work together.

It is important to pull from the power of collective behaviors because larger positive impact can be achieved for certain goals. For example, one person that is engaging in greener behaviors to benefit the natural environment will have positive effect, but when an entire collective urban area engages in greener behaviors in a coordinated manner, a much larger positive impact will benefit the natural environment.

4. Objectives for the design of a communication framework

Inter-building communication matters, but so does the way in which this communication happens. It is not simply enough to design buildings that exchange information interactively. These buildings must also use information to help them adapt to the needs of their occupants and ever-changing surrounding natural context. Yet, what should buildings do with such information? What is their objective and goal?

With an adaptable inter-building communication framework, built-environments can learn from each other. By better understanding and incorporating what works, and what does not work with occupants and surrounding natural contexts, adaptive sensory environments can adapt and improve in entirely new ways. For example, a hospital building can learn how to better personalize its healing environments by interpreting information from a home. Conversely, a home can interpret information from a hospital to help a patient recover from illness post hospital stay.

Multiple simultaneous dialogs are critical for the successful design of an inter-building communication framework. Such built-environments must not only communicate with each other, but also must exchange information with occupants and the surrounding natural environment. In reality, adaptive sensory environments become a "bridge" that adaptively re-presents nature to occupants in harmonious, beautiful, and beneficial ways.

To optimize the learning and subsequent adaptation of sensory environments, it is important for designers to engage in a "growth mindset" during design [2]. This means that building occupants, and their buildings, strive to grow and change by learning from successes as well as failures. Thus, as buildings exchange information, it becomes important for each to learn from the other by not simply replicating what the other building is doing, but by adapting their architectural behavior to their own functional needs for occupants. In other words, a hospital building that receives information from a home is not to behave exactly as a home would behave, but instead can interpret the information to improve upon its own hospital behavior. For example, a hospital can synchronize a postoperative room for improved patient sleep, but it can do this by learning specifically how to personalize the sleep environment per particular patient by learning from their home environment sleep habits.

By achieving an inter-building communication framework, it becomes possible for buildings, the natural environment, and occupants to all benefit in unique ways. For example, by coordinating efforts, a "network" of communicating buildings can pull from the power of the occupant collective to promote, sustain, and enhance green behaviors. This becomes even more empowering as buildings exchange information to work together as a team, instead of having each building work in isolation. With such inter-building communication framework designs, advancements can help to mitigate the negative effects of a changing climate.

5. Learning from human eye accommodation

The human eye holds principles by which to better understand how buildings can work together through the exchange and interpretation of information. By uncovering how the human eye focuses, a biomimetic model forms. Eye accommodation, or eye focusing, allows the eye to adapt to ever-changing object distances with the goal of seeing clearly. Similarly, the buildings that comprise a city must adapt to meet the ever-changing goals of its citizens. But how can they coordinate efforts to change their "focus" as citizen needs and goals change in real time?

Within the human eye, there are muscles that simultaneously move to allow for the expansion and contraction of the eye's lens. In essence, this muscle behavior allows for the harnessing of the lens' power, which is to focus [3]. In following this model, one can see that buildings are akin to the eye muscles, while occupants are akin to the eye lens. In other words, adaptive sensory environments can adapt to harness and enhance the power of their occupants. This can help them to coordinate efforts and achieve milestones and goals not previously possible.

Communication between buildings can foster coordination and collaboration for learning and subsequent improvement. It is important to note that adaptive sensory environments, behaving in a muscle-like manner, are able to help boost occupant efforts through both teamwork and learning. The environment can help occupants with better collaboration, which in turn, can improve learning and overall goal attainment. For example, if city citizens want to engage in greener behaviors, then communicating buildings can target and focus upon different and complementary goals including increased recycling, reduced energy consumption, and less unnecessary waste. The inter-communicating buildings act as muscles that help empower the effort of city citizens to not only support their efforts, but to also coordinate and reward them.

6. Learning from stereopsis for 3D vision

The human eyes provide an excellent example and model for how adaptive sensory buildings can communicate with one another. By studying and decoding how the biological system of the human eyes function together, architects and urban planners can expand their thinking about how to design beyond the typical boundaries within architectural and urban conditions. In particular, the eyes model how a design can work by continuously focusing on visual targets that are ever-changing, much like the real-world dynamics within which architecture and urban environments must adapt. It is by using the way human eyes coordinate as a biomimetic model that a "communication bridge" can be developed to allow for the "sensemaking" of data flowing from and to buildings so they can communicate. Just as muscles help the human eyes to focus vision, the communication bridge helps buildings to focus design behavior.

One human eye that focuses is quite powerful, but two eyes that focus simultaneously unlock the power of three-dimensional vision. Without both eyes focusing, depth of vision is not as evident. Thus, as buildings engage in communication with each other, just as two eyes do to create stereopsis; an entirely new third behavior is born. In other words, one eye focuses on an object, but both eyes can focus to see that object in perspective with depth. The same becomes true with the design of inter-communicating adaptive sensory environments. As buildings communicate, entirely new third behaviors are born.

Without inter-building communication, environments can work against one another. One building can literally undo what another has worked so hard to accomplish within a city. Similarly, a lack of stereopsis where both the eyes are not communicating with the brain as a team, can result in double vision; thus, detracting from the ultimate goal of the eyes, which is to see perspective clearly [4]. For this reason, when designers can learn from the way stereopsis works, they can begin to create urban inter-communicating environments that work together to unleash new collective building behaviors. Hence, adaptive sensory environments create a type of compound effect as can be seen in **Figure 1**.

In **Figure 1**, Building A and Building B communicate through a real-time collaboration where environmental features learn from each other to optimize building performance for goal-attainment. In essence, communicating buildings can "tune" their behaviors to guide, teach, and reward occupants as they strive to meet their goals, whether they are for an individual or for the collective. As both buildings work together to optimize their performance, a compound effect emerges as focused behaviors generate smarter citizen decision-making that

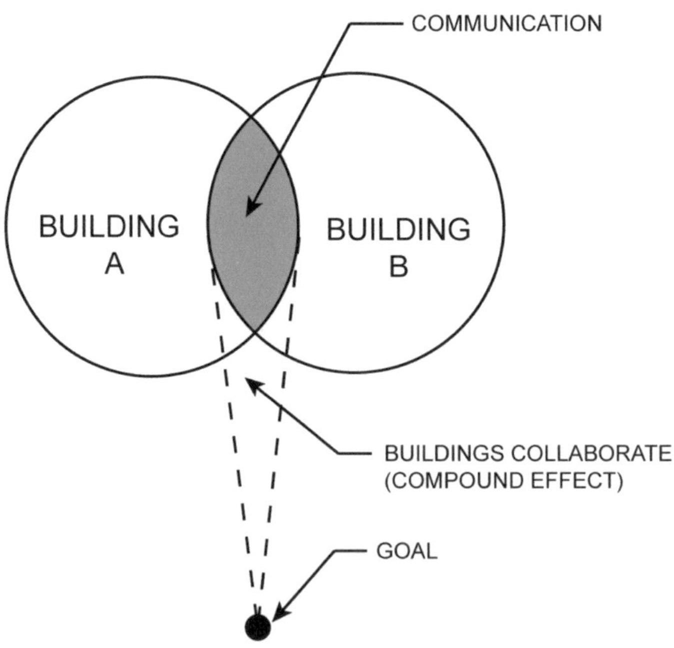

Figure 1. The compound effect of collective behaviors.

http://dx.doi.org/10.5772/intechopen.72911

positively impacts entire urban areas. Thus, a two-way dialog between buildings and occupants becomes critical as each does their part to meet a particular goal.

7. Inter-building communication to target goals in real time

Buildings that learn from each other by cooperating and collaborating make a city more nimble in responding to needs. The third behavior formed as buildings cooperate with each other means that the built-environment is not working against itself. Instead, it is harnessing its resources to yield a cumulative positive impact. In addition, as needs and goals change over time, this third behavior can be focused upon different targets because adaptive sensory buildings can change and "tune" in real time.

For example, if a city experiences a drought, citizens can work together to conserve water, "bridged" and supported by the adaptive sensory buildings. As these buildings communicate, they will nimbly optimize the way they guide, enhance, and reward city citizens. Then, as extreme weather conditions change, the city can adapt to mitigate new challenges, as these become new goals. Just as the human eyes are continuously focusing on different objects at different distances, the adaptive sensory buildings that communicate with one another can continuously adjust their aim as they target different needs and goals over time.

Inter-building communication amplifies and empowers collective occupant behaviors in real time. By using emerging technologies, such buildings can utilize social media, gamification, and even website design principles to optimize themselves with interpreted information from other buildings. These digital "doors" help adaptive sensory environments to have dialog with each other, with their occupants, and with the surrounding natural context. For example, information can be interpreted by a hospital through social media created by an individual or the collective, by recognizing winning or losing design behaviors through gamification, or by analyzing data regarding the design of different postoperative recovery rooms to see which configurations work best for a particular situation.

Thus, communication that is coordinated and collaborative is the linchpin to "focusing" or meeting ever-changing needs and goals. This becomes quite important as an overarching equilibrium point to keep the planet and occupants healthy is a primary aim, but the way in which to achieve health for the planet and occupants changes over time. Adaptability of an entire city can be harnessed through its buildings by pulling from the power of both the individual and the collective.

In **Figure 2**, one can see how buildings can work to exchange information that helps them to create a third behavior—where both occupants and buildings are working synergistically to focus on different urban needs and goals. As Building A and Building B engage with one another, the way they communicate and interpret information changes as goals shift over time. In other words, communicating buildings can collaborate in real time to meet simultaneous goals and/or shifting goals set by citizens. Buildings act as eye muscles that help occupants to focus their behaviors toward helping them reach their desired goals at micro- and macro-scales. Thus, through inter-building communication, it becomes possible to have

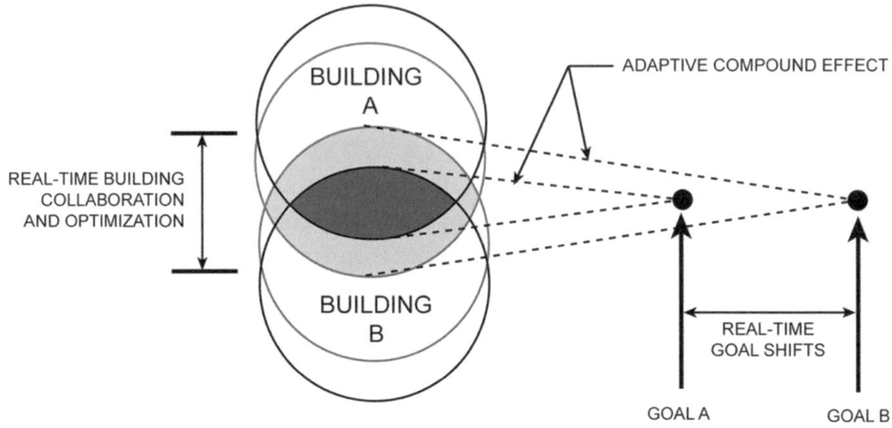

Figure 2. System design using the human eye as a model.

urban buildings work both independently and collectively for the good of both the citizen and the planet. All of this becomes possible with inter-communicating adaptive sensory environments.

8. Evoking beneficial occupant behaviors

Buildings that communicate can engage individuals to contribute beneficially through collective behaviors that achieve urban goals. Adaptive sensory environments that exchange information create a third behavior that is a hybrid behavior, which can tackle goals differently than if individual buildings never communicated. The benefit of this resides in the way such buildings can learn from each other—through designed competition, by applying tested design methods, or by learning directly from the preferences of city citizens.

For instance, inter-building communication evokes greener behavior in citizens, and thus, brings impact that is more positive to the planet. As weather has potential to become extreme, citizens need to coordinate their efforts to mitigate negative weather effects. An inter-building communication framework provides the amplifier by which citizens can pull individual efforts together to make a real difference.

An adaptive sensory environment can help its building occupants to engage in greener behaviors like recycling, using less energy, and walking or cycling instead of driving an automobile. Using gamification, it becomes possible to not only guide, enhance, and reward citizens for their greener behaviors, but it also becomes possible for the whole urban area to optimize itself as each building can adapt to incorporate design integrations that are successfully working in other buildings. Thus, the city is made up of self-optimizing buildings that work together, and not in isolation—as they learn through testing, correction, and adaptation. Citizens benefit as their usage of such buildings impacts what and how environments in such a city get optimized.

9. Creating an inter-building "communication bridge"

Creating an inter-building "communication bridge" is like seeing the city as a brain that flexes its muscles (the buildings) to focus its lenses (the occupants) to meet more collective needs faster and with higher quality. In essence, a city can mirror the plasticity of the human brain as it adjusts and changes over time to meet citizen needs and goals. The inter-building communication framework enhances such plasticity, as the third behaviors resulting from collaborating buildings allow for new kinds of evolutionary growth.

As a city works to optimize itself for its citizens, it must pull from its best features to uplift those weaker ones. As adaptive sensory environments communicate with each other, new ways in which to collaborate surface and city optimization can turn into faster and more profound evolution.

A framework for how such a city-wide inter-building communication system can be realized arises with the proliferation of nanotechnology, ubiquitous computing, wearables, micro-architectures, and the interconnection of everyday things. These sensing and data collecting devices can relay real-time data into the communication bridge. Cities can use one or multiple bridges by which to facilitate inter-building collaboration. By interpreting and correlating in-flowing data through pattern-detection methods, a "sensemaking" action occurs at the bridge, by which to make optimal city-wide decisions. From these data, building actuators can interact and engage with their occupants at more micro-levels. Thus, the communication bridge makes inter-building communication and collaboration possible (**Figure 3**).

An example of present-day technology that would help such a communication bridge to be realized can be seen in the Hexagon Geospatial Smart Maps. These smart maps create interfaces by which to visualize and assess quality and incidents of aspects like urban or building infrastructure and resources through a real-time dashboard that provides insights on conditions as they occur. Such maps have been used for the 2016 Brazil Olympics to help with real-time safety in Rio de Janeiro where the smart map interface allowed for 360-degree views

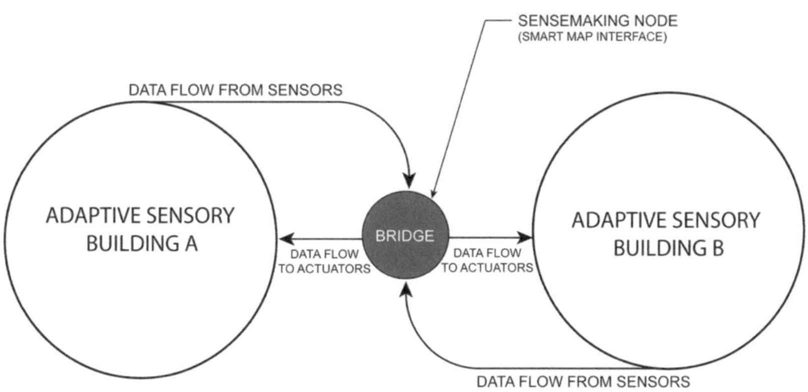

Figure 3. Inter-building communication bridge.

through a digital model of the real Olympic city along with the map interface by which to monitor and analyze incident place, time, and patterns. Again, all of this was key to help keep safety throughout the Olympic city [5]. Smart maps are also being used in the Netherlands to help assess and make decisions about infrastructure that is so critical in this location where road traffic, weather patterns, and water infrastructure must be monitored and evaluated continuously [6].

Smart maps are an example of how real-time data can be collected through sensors, analyzed, correlated, and used to make decisions not only after an event occurs, but also while it is occurring or even before it occurs (through predictive measures). With smart maps it becomes possible to engage in the sensemaking of data for building collaboration and coordination. These maps become a critical piece of the communication bridge.

Yet, the role of technology in creating an inter-building communication bridge is critical. While technology contributing to the Internet of Everything (IoE) helps to make inter-building communication possible, there are certain challenges that arise. For example, such technology should not isolate or confuse. In other words, one must beware of having a particular building or feature design become the majority that isolates or diminishes the minority [7]. In addition, inter-building communication technology should not create such complex design solutions that they become useless.

It also is important to preserve certain functions within building types that could become more hybrid. In this case, it may be beneficial to redefine building types to innovate functions that are better suited for meeting occupant needs and goals in this adaptive sensory design manner. For example, an office building may innovate its functionality by learning from a school, as it places more emphasis upon learning and free "play" time for creative thinking by workers. As such buildings communicate, new goals and priorities will arise—perhaps creativity becomes more important than productivity within certain businesses.

Furthermore, it also becomes important for adaptive sensory environments to nurture the occupant cultures they serve. In this case, a particular office building culture may be very different from another office building culture. Such inter-building communication that helps buildings optimize themselves must customize the way in which it interprets information from another building. An office building can learn from another without sacrificing what makes it unique.

In the end, inter-building communication between adaptive sensory environments is most effective when buildings learn from one another while also fusing into third behaviors that allow the city to "focus" on its prioritized citizen needs and goals.

10. The role of gamification, social media, and augmented reality

Technologies for inter-building communication frameworks give rise to such usages as gamification, social media, and augmented reality. And these all can converge to form the real-time design and optimization of place. As gamification provides incentive, guidance, and reward to occupants, social media can help such occupants to coordinate and collaborate for the common good. Augmented reality can help occupants to make more informed decisions since, with this technological advancement, they can see deeper into their environments. In this way, there will be a convergence between the digital and physical.

Just as the human eye works to form perception from physical objects, inter-building communication technologies will help occupants make smarter decisions from physical environments. These decisions can lead to greener, healthier, safer, and even more productive or creative behaviors. The guiding principle of all of this is to not only have adaptive sensory environments communicate with occupants within each building, but to also have buildings communicate with each other city-wide, so the collective of citizen behaviors can have more profound positive impact upon their future, particularly as these behaviors become smarter over time.

11. A/B split test for behavioral optimization

The brain adapts as it forms visual perceptions from what the eyes see, and this ability to compensate for visual discrepancies is very important. For example, if one eye is focusing more weakly than the other, then the brain will bias the stronger eye. Thus, a similar approach to inter-building communication can work as a healthy competition, or A/B Split Test can be used to optimize buildings in real time.

Healthy competition between buildings can work if a learning approach is at the core of the competition. An A/B Split Test, a term and practice used in website design, can be applied to inter-communicating adaptive sensory buildings. Since each building adapts to its occupants' needs and goals in real time, it is important for environments to not become design "echo chambers"—where architectural features optimize themselves in a closed loop.

In **Figure 4**, the difference between closed loop and open loop optimization can be seen. The key is to have adaptive sensory buildings interconnect through a communication network that allows collaborating building clusters to participate proactively in real-time city-wide goals. Furthermore, such a city-wide communication network can help building clusters to learn from one another. For example, one cluster may create a better A/B Split Test that can be replicated in another cluster. In the end, it is important for inter-communicating buildings to be connected for local, city, and global benefits. After all, highly successful building clusters can impact environments in different cities as they learn, interpret, and apply the positive results. An open loop design framework is vital for inter-building adaptive sensory communication.

Within an open loop design optimization of place, environments both reference themselves and other buildings outside of themselves to help them learn, adapt, and grow. This type of evolution can be empowered by adapting an A/B Split Test approach.

During a website design A/B Split Test, a webpage design element is tested against another alternative by tracking how website visitors interact with the element and page. For example, the winning design element may have the most visitor clicks.

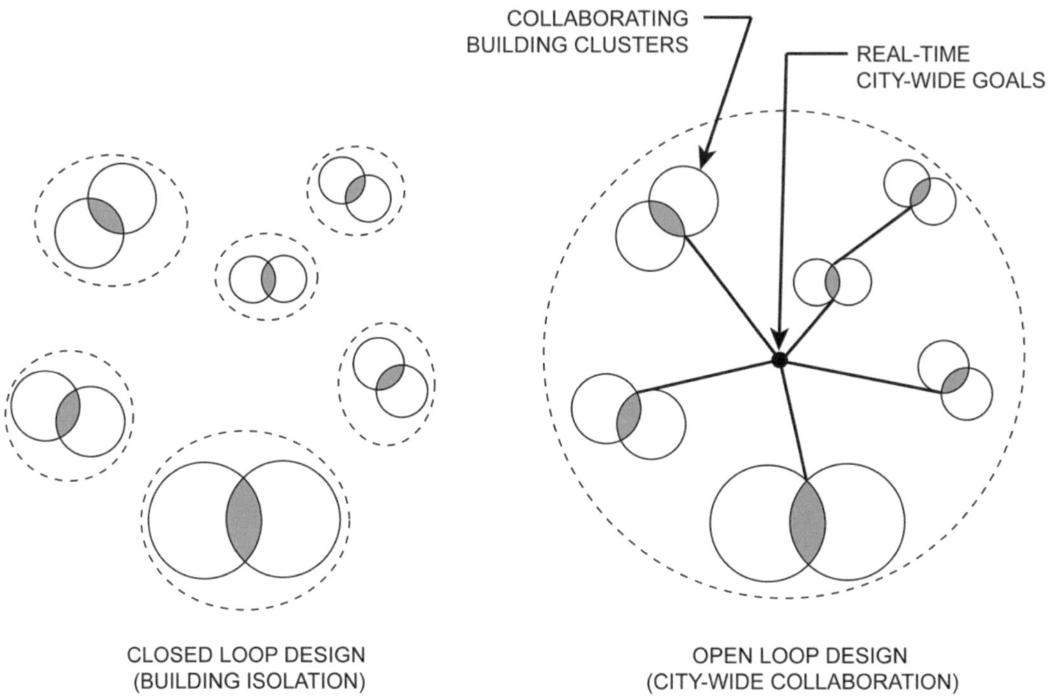

Figure 4. Closed loop versus open loop design optimization.

A/B Split Testing can be used to help encourage the positive learning and growth of inter-communicating adaptive sensory design buildings. By allowing two or even three buildings to enter into such an A/B Split Test, particular design elements can be compared against one another to see which performs best. And since these sensory buildings adapt in real time, the winning design element can be interpreted and then incorporated to optimize the other designs.

Within an A/B Split Test, design features from one hospital can be compared against another hospital's feature. Or a hospital feature in a postoperative recovery room can be compared against a patient's home bedroom. In this case, the hospital room can better "tune" as it adapts itself to optimize for ideal patient healing.

Such A/B Split Tests can be used for any building type, as long as there is a network for the inter-building communication system. In essence, Split Tests can help buildings to improve themselves by not being so self-referential. At the city scale, this allows buildings to learn from each other, and at the global scale this allows cities to collaborate.

12. Competition for growth and healing

By learning from other buildings, adaptive sensory environments can grow, as they evolve into better forms of themselves. However, they may also be able to heal themselves in real time, at a multitude of scales—from building-scale to urban-scale.

Similarly, healthy competition can be used within one building as rooms can also learn from one another. Essentially, the inter-building communication system allows environments to optimize—by reaching out to distinctly separate other environments, be they right around the corner within the city, or within another city across the globe.

The human eyes cooperate with one another, and their "competing" views are actually very critical to how the human brain and mind work to form perspective and perception. Similarly, as two buildings compete with one another, they are simply offering alternative design solutions.

It is important to note that just because building designs may be involved in an A/B Split Test, the winning design is not necessarily the better overall design. Two buildings can learn from one another, as one environment may perform better with certain functions, while another environment performs better with other functions. Inter-building communication allows for the best design integrations to influence others.

The A/B Split Testing method is not a means by which designs should simply copy other designs. The interpretation of design usage in one place can influence the way a design operates in another. However, care should be taken to ensure that a place does not lose its authenticity.

As inter-building communication unifies city buildings through form, function, and even meaning, it becomes important for the authenticity of place to remain standing. After all, the certain culture of a particular office building, or the way a hospital nurtures its patients in a particular part of the world will likely differ. Yet, universal lessons can be learned, interpreted, and applied from building to building within different cultures.

By using healthy competition to improve designs in real time, larger leaps in design evolution can be taken. Adaptive sensory environments that communicate with each other become innovators, driven by the thumbprint of their original architectural designers.

In the end, such healthy competition helps to strengthen what works, and helps to eliminate design weaknesses. This is particularly advantageous as certain citizen goals surface. The aim of A/B Split Testing environments through inter-building communication is to find those key leverage points where optimal benefit can be pulled from a design to positively impact more people. Yet, healthy competition is only one way in which to use the system framework of inter-building communication.

As buildings advance in the way they are able to communicate and learn from each other, greater occupant customization will become possible through occupant control points. For example, an occupant can "bridge" their home office preferences with their office building workplace preferences—to either keep them different or similar. The key with inter-building communication is to allow personal choice for occupants when they need it, while also being versatile enough as a design to be able to present them with those choices.

As environmental designs learn from each other, the choices and variations they can provide occupants for certain situations will grow as well. Thus, buildings will be better able to adapt, to nurture, and to grow with the occupants they serve. This will strengthen design so as to help it "fit" occupants at a more nuanced level. Again, this will help them to learn better, to make smarter decisions better, and to engage in more beneficial behaviors.

13. The emergence of symbiotic ecosystems

As inter-building communication links buildings together into a type of network, an ecosystem emerges. Much like the natural environment ecosystem, the city ecosystem cultivates the power to heal itself, particularly as buildings use such information "bridges" to learn from each other. And when both urban and natural ecosystems interact adaptively with one another, they become symbiotic.

By using teamwork at all scales: rooms within buildings learn from each other to optimize a building, buildings within cities learn from each other to optimize a city, and cities within the world can learn from each other to optimize for global goals. All of this teamwork can be thought of as an important collective "challenge" with missions that serve different scales.

As buildings work together through learning and adapting, they help to empower and enhance citizen efforts to improve their own individual quality of life, and the collective quality of life that serves the greater good. Similarly, the eyes that help the human body to see empower the person to improve their quality of life in new ways. In other words, citizens are the lenses of the city—giving the city focus through adapting buildings that work to meet goals by acting collaboratively.

In essence, the built-environment ecosystem can enter into a new type of dialog with the natural environment ecosystem. This symbiotic relationship serves to help each ecosystem enhance, grow, and heal itself. For example, as cities harness built-environment and citizen behaviors, they can positively impact the natural environment by adapting or even reversing disturbances.

Inter-building communication for adaptive sensory environments is key to magnifying the positive effects of beneficial behaviors. As the built and natural ecosystems enter into a two-way dialog, architectural design will keep occupants at the center, but in additional new ways. Inter-building communication extends the reach of beneficial citizen behaviors, while also pulling from these behaviors to harmonize with nature anew.

By strategically designing inter-building communication within cities, a renewed relationship between the built and natural worlds arises. This way of designing will raise the consciousness of citizens so they engage in smarter decision-making while also knowing that their behaviors have a tangible impact upon the greater context that is the planet. Thus, buildings can be designed to communicate so they can retain their individual authenticity but can also act together to create maximized positive impact.

Just as the eyes see to help a person visualize where they are going, with communication, the city can "see" to help citizens visualize where they are going. Furthermore, as inter-building communication is applied to adaptive sensory environments, those citizens will have the ability to optimize, enhance, and take action on behaviors that lead to their goals—including a safer environment, a healthier planet, and a happier world.

http://dx.doi.org/10.5772/intechopen.72911

Author details

Maria Lorena Lehman

Address all correspondence to: mll@sensingarchitecture.com

MLL Design Lab, LLC, Sensing Architecture® Academy, Massachusetts, United States

References

[1] Lehman ML. Adaptive Sensory Environments. Oxon/New York: Routledge; 2017. p. 1

[2] Dweck CS. Mindset: The New Psychology of Success. New York: Ballantine Books; 2008. pp. 3-14

[3] Nave R. HyperPhysics: Accommodation. [Internet]. 2016. Available from: http://hyperphysics.phy-astr.gsu.edu/hbase/vision/accom.html [Accessed: Mar 29, 2017]

[4] Ang B. Vision and Eye Health: Stereopsis. [Internet]. 2017. Available from: http://www.vision-and-eye-health.com/stereopsis.html [Accessed: Mar 29, 2017]

[5] Hexagon Geospatial. Hexagon Smart City Rio Project. [Internet]. 2016. Available from: https://www.youtube.com/watch?v=YtOoLovYZZo [Accessed: Oct 11, 2017]

[6] Hexagon Geospatial. Making Smart Cities in the Netherlands. [Internet]. 2016. Available from: https://www.youtube.com/watch?v=q1gbzJQfv2c [Accessed: Oct 11, 2017]

[7] Johnson S. Emergence. New York: Scribner; 2001. p. 161

Chapter 3

Taking Inspiration from Flying Insects to Navigate inside Buildings

Julien R. Serres

Additional information is available at the end of the chapter

http://dx.doi.org/10.5772/intechopen.72918

Abstract

These days, flying insects are seen as genuinely agile micro air vehicles fitted with smart sensors and also parsimonious in their use of brain resources. They are able to visually navigate in unpredictable and GPS-denied environments. Understanding how such tiny animals work would help engineers to figure out different issues relating to drone miniaturization and navigation inside buildings. To turn a drone of ~1 kg into a robot, miniaturized conventional avionics can be employed; however, this results in a loss of their flight autonomy. On the other hand, to turn a drone of a mass between ~1 g (or less) and ~500 g into a robot requires an innovative approach taking inspiration from flying insects both with regard to their flapping wing propulsion system and their sensory system based mainly on motion vision in order to avoid obstacles in three dimensions or to navigate on the basis of visual cues. This chapter will provide a snapshot of the current state of the art in the field of bioinspired optic flow sensors and optic flow-based direct feedback loops applied to micro air vehicles flying inside buildings.

Keywords: optic flow, sense and avoid system, micro air vehicle (MAV), unmanned aerial vehicle (UAV), bionics, bioinspired robotics

1. Introduction

1.1. The biorobotic approach

Fifty years ago, Karl von Frisch observed that foraging bees fly to a distance somewhat greater than 13 km from their hive in search of food sources [1], but honeybees were not able to be trained to collect a reward beyond this limit; it thus corresponded to their maximum foraging distance. The area of the circle, whose center is the hive and radius the maximum foraging distance, represents a huge surface area of 530 km^2. Even knowing that the average length of a honeybee is about 13 mm, the volume of its brain is lower than 1 mm^3 and contains around 960,000 neurons [2, 3], and each worker honeybee's compound eye contains ~5500 facets comprised of nine photosensitive cells (i.e., 99,000 photosensitive cells for the whole worker bee's visual system) [4]; it is still unknown what visual cues are used during honeybees' journeys nor how they are used in flight to recognize its location and to navigate within a space whose dimensions are a million times larger than their bodies. Karl von Frisch was awarded the Nobel Prize in Physiology or Medicine 1973 for his scientific achievement in describing the honeybees' "waggle dance," which is used by bees to communicate both the distance and the azimuthal orientation of a profitable nectar source. The 8-shaped geometry of the waggle dance codes the position of a nectar source. The duration of the waggle is closely correlated to the distance of the nectar source [5], and the honeybee's odometer appears to be driven by motion vision [6]. The "8" orientation is highly correlated to the azimuthal orientation of a nectar source [1]. In flight, honeybees use a kind of "solar compass" based on polarized ultraviolet light [7–9] instead of a "magnetic compass" to maintain their heading toward the nectar source or their hive. Karl von Frisch therefore concluded that bees "recruited" by this dance used the information encoded in it to guide them directly to the remote food source. To better understand the honeybee's recruitment process, the Biorobotics Lab at the Freie Universität Berlin has developed a robotic honeybee mimicking the "waggle dance" using a biorobotic approach [10].

While the biological substrate has not yet been fully identified [12], the biorobotic approach is particularly useful both in the fields of neuroscience and robotics [13–20], because the robotic model can be tested under similar experimental conditions such as ethological experiments and it can suggest new biological hypotheses (**Figure 1**). From these interactions between ethological experiments, computational models, and robotics (**Figure 1**), uncertainties can be removed by considering the minimum requirements to perform any navigational tasks (e.g., [21–25]). Insect-sized micro air vehicles (MAVs) are increasingly becoming a reality [26–31] and in the future will have to be fitted with sensors and flight control devices enabling them to perform all kinds of aerial maneuvers inside buildings including takeoff, floor, ceiling and wall avoidance, tunnel-following, and landing.

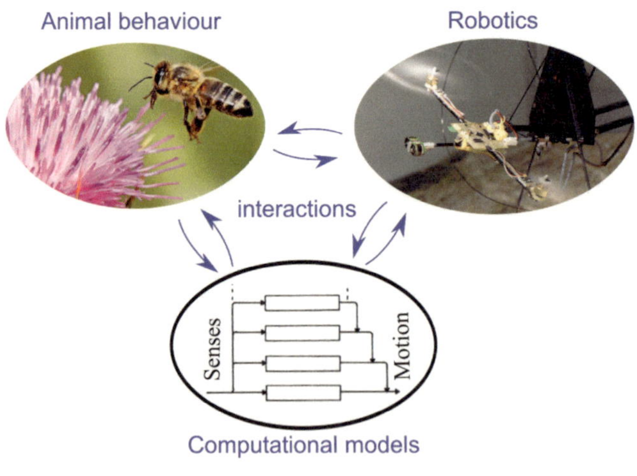

Figure 1. Description of the biorobotic approach using successive interactions between animal behavior, computational models, and robotics. Picture of the honeybee landing on a milk thistle flower from Wikimedia commons (picture taken by Fir0002/Flagstaffotos under CC-BY license). Picture of the BeeRotor robot fitted with a twin CurvACE artificial compound eye from [11] under CC-BY license.

1.2. What is optic flow?

The optic flow perceived by an agent (an animal, a robot, or a human) is particularly dependent on the structure of the environment [32–36]. Optic flow can be defined by a vector field of the apparent angular velocity of objects, surfaces, and edges in a visual scene caused by the relative motion between an agent and the scene (**Figure 2**). Optic flow $\vec{\omega}$ (Eq. (1)) is the combination of two optic flow components: a translational optic flow $\vec{\omega}_T$ and a rotational optic flow $\vec{\omega}_R$ [35]:

$$\vec{\omega} = \vec{\omega}_T + \vec{\omega}_R \tag{1}$$

Flying insects like hymenopterans stabilize their heads by compensating for any body rotations [37]. Accordingly, any robot's visual system is assumed to be perfectly stabilized in space, therefore canceling all rotation due to body pitch and roll with respect to the inertial frame. Consequently, the robot's visual system experiences only translational optic flow, and the visual system will receive a purely translational optic flow ($\vec{\omega}_R = \vec{0}$). The translational optic flow (expressed in rad/s) can be defined as follows:

$$\vec{\omega}_T = -\frac{\vec{V} - \left(\vec{V} \cdot \vec{d}\right) \cdot \vec{d}}{D\left(\vec{d}\right)} \tag{2}$$

where $\vec{d}$ is a unit vector describing the viewing direction, $\vec{V}$ is the translational velocity vector and $D\left(\vec{d}\right)$ is the distance from the object as seen by photosensors.

However, in the horizontal plane, the magnitude of the translational optic flow, which describes the front-to-back motion occurring when the agent moves forward, depends only on the ratio between the relative linear speed V and the distance D_φ from the objects providing an optical contrast in the environment (the walls in **Figure 2**) and the azimuth angle φ between the gaze direction and the speed vector (Eq. (3)):

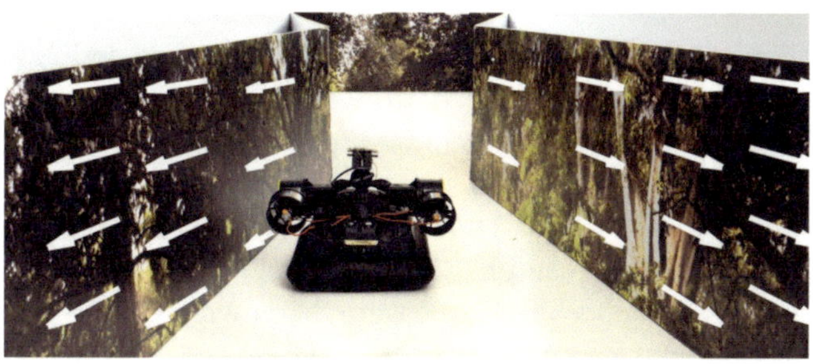

Figure 2. The LORA robot fitted with a heading-lock system travels straightforward through a tapered corridor perceiving a purely translational optic flow. This optic flow experienced by the robot is schematized by the white arrows (i.e., angular velocity vectors) on the walls (adapted from [25] under CC-BY license).

$$\omega_T = \frac{V}{D_\varphi} \cdot \sin(\varphi) \tag{3}$$

Translational optic flow (Eq. (3)) is particularly appropriate for short-range navigation because it depends on the ratio between (i) the relative linear speed of an object in the scene with respect to the agent and (ii) the distance from obstacles in the surrounding environment: this visual angular speed cue does not require either speed or distance measurement (Eq. (3)).

1.3. Why use optic flow in robotics?

Flying robots are today capable of accurately evaluating their pose in outdoor flight using conventional sensors such as the global positioning system (GPS) and inertial measurement unit (IMU). This is very efficient for long-range navigation at hundreds of meters above the ground, without any obstacles around, for example, an airplane in cruising flight. Nevertheless, the expanding set of roles for flying robots increasingly calls for them to operate close to obstacles (<1 m) in all directions in GPS-denied or cluttered environments including buildings, warehouses, performance halls, or urban canyons. Robots can have difficulties receiving the GPS signal, but they have to pick up the 3D structure of the surrounding environment to avoid obstacles and accomplish their missions. At such a short distance from obstacles (<1 m), the environment is completely unpredictable: it is obviously very difficult to map the entire environment in 3D at such a scale in real time. A more efficient approach would consist of the robot continuously using local information to avoid obstacles while waiting for global information to pursue its mission. Most of the time, the use of emissive proximity sensors such as ultrasonic or laser range finders, radar, or scanning light detection and ranging (LIDAR) has been considered for this purpose. Such emissive sensors can be bulky, stealth-compromising, high energy, and low-bandwidth, compromising their utility for tiny and insect-like robots [26–31]. It is well known that flying insects are sensitive to optic flow [16, 19, 36, 38]; moreover, they are able to measure the optic flow of their surroundings irrespective of the spatial texture and contrast [39, 40] and also that some of their neurons respond monotonically to optic flow [36, 41]. Consequently, there are considerable benefits in terms of both number of pixels and computational resources by designing guidance systems for micro flying robots fitted with passive sensing, such as motion vision, inspired by flying insects.

1.4. The chicken-and-egg problem of translational optic flow

A given magnitude of translational optic flow is a kind of chicken-and-egg problem (Eq. (3)), because an infinite number of couples (speed; distance) lead to the same speed/distance ratio, in other words the same optic flow magnitude, coming from a surface (**Figure 3a**). For instance, an optic flow magnitude of 2 rad/s (i.e., 115°/s) can be generated by a robot flying at 1 m/s at 0.5 m above the floor, flying at 2 m/s at 1 m above the floor, and so on (**Figure 3a**). To get around the optic flow chicken-and-egg problem, roboticists introduced the assumption prevailing in those days that robots have to measure their own speed by using a tachymeter on wheels [21, 42], a GPS unit [43], or a custom-built Pitot tube [44], in order to assess the distance from obstacles and then to avoid them, and conversely have to measure the distance from obstacle by means of an ultrasonic distance sensor [45] in order to assess their own ground speed. However, flying insects are not able to directly measure their true ground speed (but

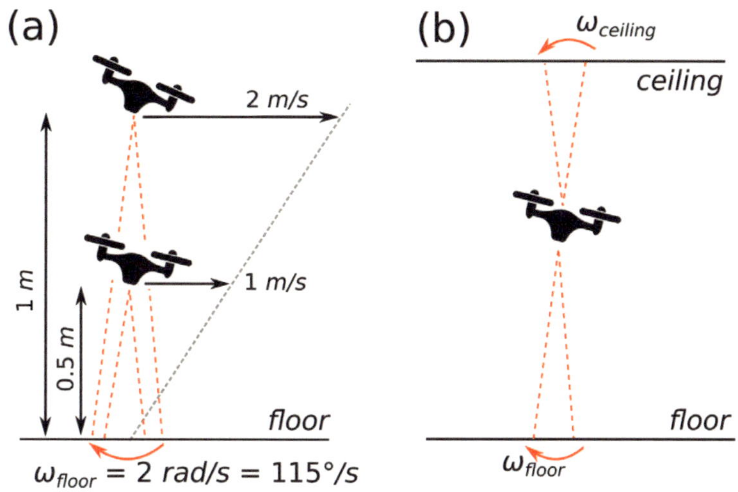

Figure 3. (a) The chicken-and-egg problem of translational optic flow. An infinite number of couples (speed; distance) lead to the same speed/distance ratio ω_{ground} (the same angular velocity/optic flow magnitude). For instance, in this illustration an optic flow magnitude of $\omega_{ground} = 2$ rad/s (or 115°/s) is coming from the ground. (b) To get around the optic flow chicken-and-egg problem shown in (a), the flying agent has to pick up optic flow in a wide field of view or in different parts of the field of view, here by jointly measuring optic flow coming from the ceiling ($\omega_{ceiling}$) and the floor (ω_{floor}).

only their airspeed [46] or their airspeed rate [38]) or their distance from obstacles by using their binocular vision which is too limited [47]. Flying insects do not actually solve the optic flow chicken-and-egg problem to cross tunnels but instead use visuomotor feedback loops directly based on optic flow by perceiving it in a wide field of view with their compound eyes seeing both the floor and the ceiling (**Figure 3b**) and also the walls [48, 49].

2. Bioinspired optic flow sensors

The criteria for evaluation of the potential of optic flow sensors for MAV applications include:

- Visual sensors must be able to deal with the large dynamic range of natural irradiance levels, which can cover up to 9 decades during the course of the day.
- Range of optic flow covered (i.e., the angular speed magnitude), defined by the number of optic flow decades. There is now evidence that flying insects are able to measure the optic flow over a range of more than 1.4 decades [41, 50].
- Accuracy and precision, defined by systematic errors and coefficients of variation $C_V < 0.5$.
- Output refresh rate, defined by the instantaneous output frequency (>10 Hz).

2.1. Taking inspiration from the compound eye

The structure of a compound eye is based on a large number of repeating units called ommatidia (**Figure 4**). Each ommatidia is composed of a facet (hexagonal lens, diameter from ~30 to

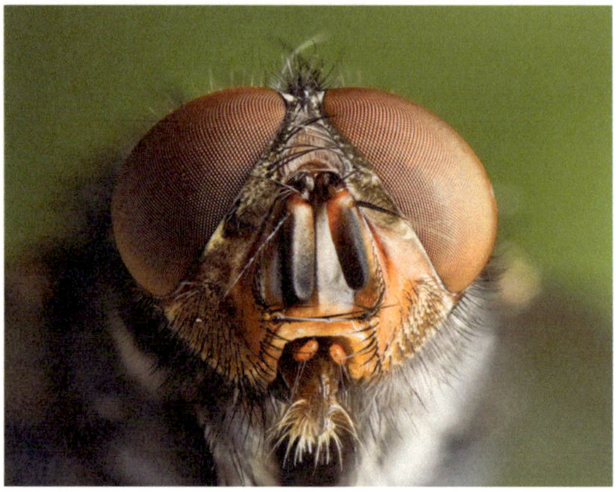

Figure 4. Head of a blue bottle fly *Calliphora vomitoria,* Austin's ferry, Tasmania, Australia (2009). Picture: J.J. Harisson under CC-BY license. There are 6000 ommatidia per compound eye of a blowfly *Calliphora erythrocephala*. The two compound eyes cover 85% of the visual field, which represents a full panoramic view field except in their blind spot caused by their own body. The minimum interommatidial angle of a *Calliphora erythrocephala* visual system is $\Delta\Phi = 1.1^{\circ}$ in the frontal part, up to 2° in the ventral part [52].

~60 μm) which focuses the incoming light toward the photosensitive cells [19, 51]. Each ommatidia optical axis is separated by an interommatidial angle $\Delta\phi$ which defines the spatial acuity of the visual system [52]. The interommatidial angles $\Delta\phi$ are smaller in the frontal part of the visual system than in the lateral, dorsal, or ventral parts as observed in any compound eye [52–54]. In bioinspired robots, a sine-law gradient (Eq. (4)) is generally used in the horizontal plane in artificial compound eye design [21]:

$$\Delta\phi(\varphi) = \Delta\phi(90^{\circ}) \cdot \sin(\varphi) \tag{4}$$

Once the spatial sampling has been carried out, the narrowness of the ommatidia performs a type of automatic low-pass filtering on the visual signals reaching the photosensitive cells. The diffraction of the light through the lens leads to a Gaussian angular sensitivity [52, 55, 56], which acts as a blurring effect. This angular sensitivity is described by the width at half height, called the acceptance angle $\Delta\rho$ (Eq. (5)):

$$\Delta\rho = \sqrt{\frac{\lambda}{D_l} + \frac{D_r}{f}} \tag{5}$$

where D_l is the lens diameter, λ is the wavelength, D_r is the rhabdom diameter (i.e., pixel diameter in artificial design), and f is the ommatidium focal length. The acceptance angle $\Delta\rho$ and the interommatidial angle are roughly equal ($\Delta\rho \approx \Delta\phi$) in diurnal insects [52] for each ommatidium, which allows for continuity in visual signals (low aliasing) and avoids oversampling the environment. Moreover, the photosensitive cells' dynamics can achieve a temporal frequency up to 100 Hz in dipterans [57]; well beyond human vision (central vision up to 50 Hz).

In artificial design, most of the time $D_l \gg \lambda$, the light diffraction is therefore not considered; thus, $\Delta\phi = \frac{d}{f}$ with d the pixels pitch and f the focal length and $\Delta\rho \approx \Delta\phi$ can be obtained by slightly defocusing the lens (see section 2.2.). Two artificial compound eyes have been already built with either inorganic semiconductor photoreceptors comprising 630 pixels with $\Delta\phi = \Delta\rho = 4.2^{\circ}$ [58] or organic photodiodes comprising 256 pixels with $\Delta\phi = 11^{\circ}$ and $\Delta\rho = 9.7^{\circ}$ [59].

2.2. Taking inspiration from biological signal processing

Thirty years ago, a bioinspired local motion sensor (LMS) was designed [60, 61], the signal processing scheme of which was based on a time-of-travel algorithm directly inspired from fly's motion-sensitive neurons [19, 51, 62]. A time-of-travel algorithm directly measures the delay Δt taken by a contrast edge to travel between the visual axes of two adjacent pixels, separated by an inter-pixel angle $\Delta\phi$. The optic flow is therefore naturally an inverse function of this delay Δt (Eq. 6), and the optic flow range measurement depends jointly on the choice of the inter-pixel angle $\Delta\phi$ and on the timespan, which was reported from 10 to 230 ms in fly's motion-sensitive neurons [19, 51, 62] and considered in the LMS signal processing as well:

$$\omega_{meas} = \frac{\Delta\phi}{\Delta t} \tag{6}$$

The signal processing scheme of the bioinspired LMS is depicted in **Figure 5a** and can be broken down into the eight following steps:

1. Spatial sampling realized by the photoreceptor's optical axes separated by an angle $\Delta\phi$ [52, 55, 56].

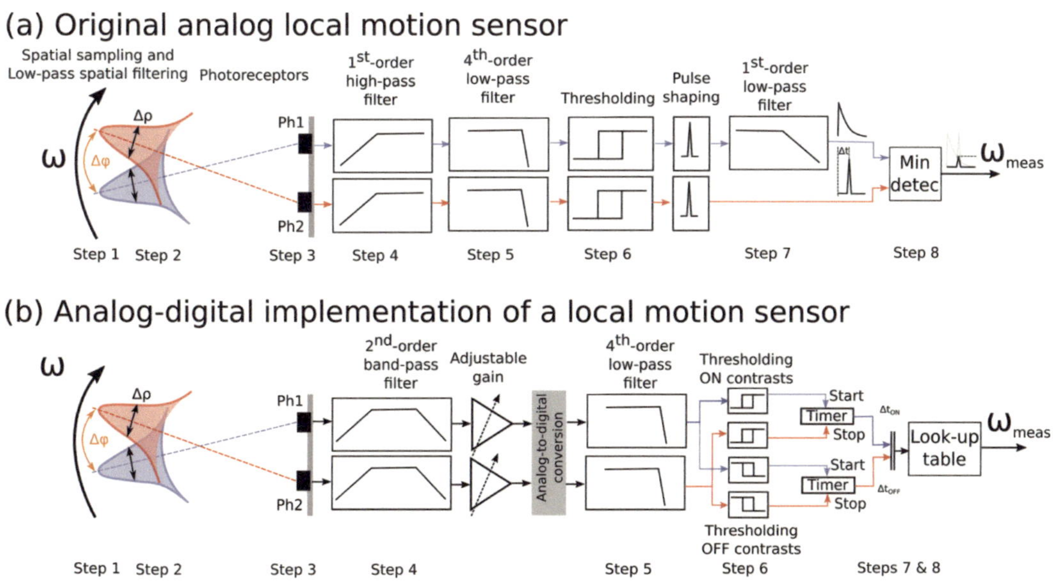

Figure 5. (a) Original analog local motion sensor (LMS). Only the thresholding stage of the ON contrast pathway is represented here, but both ON and OFF contrast pathways were implemented in the original full analog LMS in [61] (redrawn from [19]). (b) Analog-digital implementation of a local motion sensor (redrawn from [25, 63]).

2. Spatial low-pass filtering performed by the Gaussian angular sensitivity function of the defocused lens (correspond to a blurring effect) and characterized by the angular width at half height, called the acceptance angle $\Delta\rho$. Unlike natural compound eyes in which spatial low-pass filtering automatically results from diffraction [52], the cutoff spatial frequency depends on the amount of defocusing [60, 61].

3. Phototransduction: a logarithmic amplifier was originally used (five decades of lighting) [60, 61], a linear amplifier was used (three decades of lighting) [64], or more recently auto-adaptive photodetectors were designed as artificial retinas [58, 65], which consisted of a logarithmic amplifier associated with a high-gain negative feedback loop (seven decades of lighting). Results with auto-adaptive pixels are reminiscent of analogous experiments carried out on single vertebrate [66] and invertebrate [67] photodetectors.

4. Temporal high-pass filtering of photoreceptor signals in each channel not only to cancel the direct component but also to accentuate the transient signals created by contrasting edges (derivative effect).

5. Temporal low-pass filtering to reduce noise (e.g., 100 Hz interference originating from artificial lighting). Such temporal band-pass filtering was identified in two large monopolar cells L1 and L2 inside the fly's lamina [68–70]. However, two discrepancies can be reported in the technological design: the high-pass and low-pass filters are switched with respect to the biological model in the bioinspired LMS due to electronic constraints, and the low-pass filter is the fourth order in the bioinspired LMS rather than the third order in the biological model.

6. Hysteresis thresholding performed on signals to detect contrast transition and also to discriminate ON and OFF transitions. There is now strong evidence that the fly's motion pathway is fed by separate ON and OFF pathways [51, 71, 72].

7. Pulse generation on the first channel though a low-pass filter, then generating a long-lived decaying signal (first-order unit impulse response) approximating a mathematical inverse function [60, 61].

8. Pulse generation on the second channel, sampling the long-lived decaying signal coming from the first channel through a diode minimum detector circuit [60, 61]. The LMS output is therefore a pulse-shaped signal whose magnitude represents the local optic flow magnitude.

Accordingly, the optic flow measurement ω_{meas} (here in volts) results from sampling the long-lived exponentially decaying function (with a time constant τ), varies inversely with Δt, and hence increases with the true optic flow ω according to the following equation:

$$\omega_{meas}(\omega) = V_{cc} \cdot e^{-\frac{\omega_0}{\omega}} \tag{7}$$

$$\omega_0 = \frac{\Delta\phi}{\tau} \tag{8}$$

with V_{cc} representing the power supply voltage. This original analog functional scheme can measure the optic flow in a range $\left[\frac{\omega_0}{4}, 4 \cdot \omega_0\right]$, corresponding to a 1.2 decade of optic flow measurement.

This bioinspired LMS (**Figure 5**) features three major benefits: firstly, the LMS output responds monotonically to the magnitude of the optic flow and therefore acts like a local optic flow sensor, which is vital to get non-equivocal information about the distance from surrounding obstacles; secondly, the refresh rate of the LMS output is asynchronous and relatively high (>10 Hz depending on lighting conditions) which is suitable for indoor navigation; and, thirdly, the thresholding stage makes the LMS output virtually independent of texture and contrast.

The bioinspired LMS scheme based on a time-of-travel algorithm (**Figure 5**) is not a "correlator scheme" or "Hassenstein-Reichardt detector" (HR detector) [73, 74] whose output is dependent on texture and contrast. Another variant of the bioinspired LMS based on a time-of travel algorithm has been proposed over the past 20 years and is known as "facilitate-and-sample" algorithm [75, 76].

2.3. Local motion sensors and artificial retinas

Since the original analog design depicted in **Figure 5a** [60, 61], various versions of the bioinspired LMS have been built including analog-digital implementations as depicted in **Figure 5b** (for an FPAA implementation and an 8-bit microcontroller implementation running at 1 kHz [77], for an FPGA implementation running at 2.5 or 5 kHz [78], for an LTCC implementation running at 1 kHz [25, 79, 80], and for a 16-bit microcontroller implementation running at 2 kHz) [64]. These various versions of the bioinspired LMS have been built in order to reduce size, mass, or power consumption while benefiting from computational resources to increase the number of LMSs.

An original LMS version was developed including an iC-Haus™ LSC 12-channel photosensor array forming 6 pixel and five LMSs [63]. The outputs of five LMS were associated to a step merging based on a median filter; both the precision and the accuracy in the optic flow measurement were greatly improved [63]. Moreover, to increase by at least four times the number of LMSs that can be embedded in a 16-bit microcontroller, a linear interpolation applied to photosensor signals was used to reduce the sampling rate and thus save computational resources [81]. The best trade-off between computational load and accuracy was found at a sampling rate of 200 Hz [81].

In the framework of a European project called CurvACE (2009–2013; www.curvace.org), aiming at mimicking the *Drosophila melanogaster*'s compound eye, the first artificial compound eye was built [58]. This functional prototype with its 630 pixels (forming 630 artificial ommatidia) offered a wide view field ($180 \times 60°$) over a significant range of lighting conditions and weights ~2 g [58] (see twin CurvACE version in **Figure 8a**).

A recent optic flow sensor based on the M^{2}APix retina (M^{2}APix stands for Michaelis–Menten auto-adaptive pixel [65]) can auto-adapt in a 7 decade of lighting range and responds appropriately to step changes up to ± 3 decades [82]. The pixels do not saturate thanks to the normalization process performed by the very large-scale integration (VLSI) transistors [65]; this is due to the intrinsic properties of the Michaelis–Menten equation [66]. A comparison of the characteristics of auto-adaptive Michaelis–Menten and Delbrück pixels [83] under identical lighting conditions (i.e., integrated in the same retina) demonstrated better performance of the Michaelis–Menten pixels in terms of dynamic sensitivity and minimum contrast detection [65].

Different kinds of algorithms have been developed to compute local motion; these have produced different hardware implementations including templates, time of travel, feature tracking, edge counting, edge correlation, and the Hassenstein-Reichardt correlator [30, 84, 85] and also different software implementations [85]. However, analog VLSI motion sensors provide significant reductions in power consumption and payload while increasing bandwidth, improving both precision and accuracy in optic flow measurement for MAV applications.

3. Optic flow-based navigation inside buildings

3.1. Obstacle avoidance in the horizontal plane

3.1.1. Keeping the bilateral optic flow constant: a speed control system

The idea of introducing a speed control system based on optic flow was firstly developed by Coombs and Roberts [86]. Their Bee-Bot adjusted its forward speed to keep the optic flow within a measurable range, using a bilateral optic flow criterion to control the robot's speed. The bilateral optic flow criterion (sum of the left and right optic flows) as a feedback signal to directly control the robot's speed was first introduced by Santos-Victor and colleagues [87] onboard the Robee robot. Qualitatively, the robot's speed was scaled by the level of the environment's visual clutter. Since then, the bilateral optic flow criterion as a feedback signal to directly control the robot's forward speed has been tested on many robots in both straight and tapered corridors [25, 87–94]. The desired bilateral optic flow was ~12°/s for the Bee-Bot robot [87], ~19°/s in [88], ~46°/s in [88], ~21°/s in [91], 190, or 250°/s in [25] and [94]. The higher the desired bilateral optic flow, the faster the robot will advance while moving close to the walls.

3.1.2. Dual optic flow regulation

The first optic flow regulator was originally developed for ground avoidance when following terrain [25, 95]. An optic flow set point is compared to a measured optic flow to provide an error signal, this latter feeding into a regulator controlling a force orthogonal to the direction of motion. The combination of a unilateral optic flow regulator for controlling the lateral positioning on either side and a bilateral optic flow regulator for controlling the forward speed has been called a dual optic flow regulator [96]. The dual optic flow regulator concept was originally developed for aerial vehicles endowed with natural roll and pitch stabilization abilities, in which planar flight control systems can be developed conveniently [96] in order to mimic honeybees' abilities in the horizontal plane [16, 39, 97, 98] and to avoid the weaknesses of the optic flow balance strategy in the presence of lateral openings (see review [99]). The dual optic flow regulator was implemented for the first time onboard an 878-gram fully actuated hovercraft called LORA, which stands for *lateral optic flow regulator autopilot* [25, 94] (**Figure 7a**). The dual optic flow regulator is based on:

i. A unilateral optic flow regulator (**Figure 6b**) that adjusts the hovercraft's lateral thrust so as to keep the two perceived lateral optic flows higher (left or right) equal to a sideways optic flow set point (noted $\omega_{setSide}$). The outcome is that the distance to the nearest wall becomes proportional to the hovercraft's forward speed V_f, as determined in (ii).

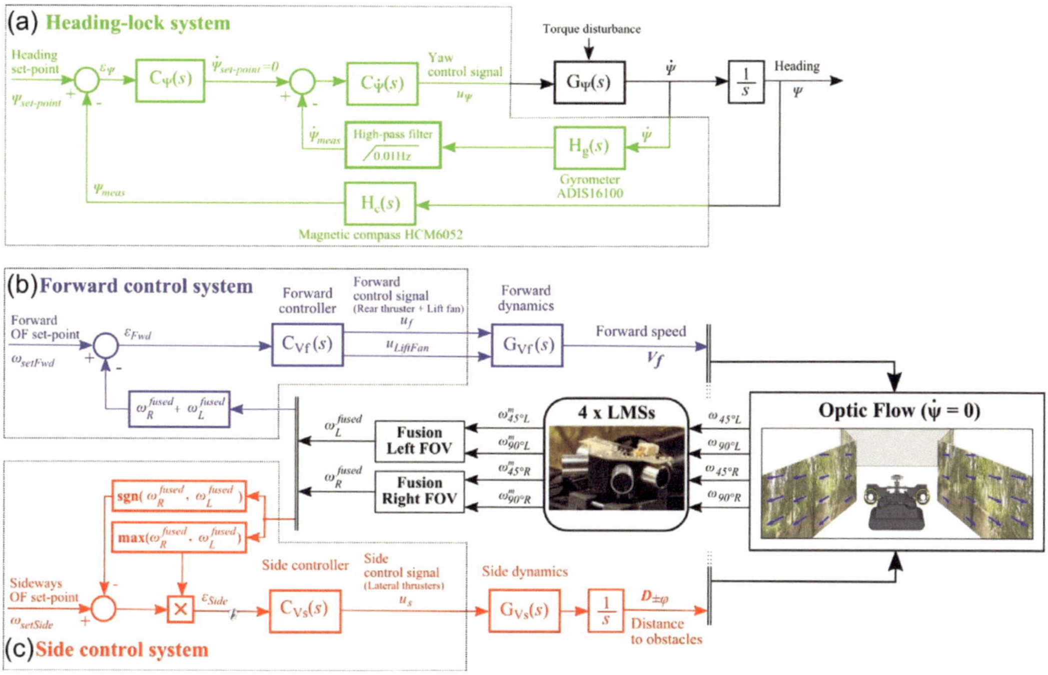

Figure 6. Functional diagram of the dual optic flow regulator (OF stands for optic flow; FOV stands for field of view; and LMS stands for local motion sensor). (a) Heading-lock system canceling any robot rotations. (b) Speed control system based on bilateral optic flow regulation. (c) Lateral obstacle system based on unilateral optic flow regulation. (from [25] under CC-BY license).

ii. A bilateral optic flow regulator (**Figure 6c**) adjusts the hovercraft's forward thrust so as to keep the sum of the two lateral optic flows (right and left) equal to a forward optic flow set point (noted ω_{setFwd}).

In a steady state, with a given corridor width of D, the final operating point of the dual optic flow regulator will be

$$V_{f\infty} = \frac{\omega_{setSide} \cdot (\omega_{setFwd} - \omega_{setSide})}{\omega_{setFwd}} \cdot D \tag{9}$$

$$y_{\infty} = \frac{\omega_{setFwd} - \omega_{setSide}}{\omega_{setFwd}} \cdot D \tag{10}$$

As a consequence, the robot's speed will asymptotically and automatically be scaled by the corridor width or even by the environment clutter (**Figure 7b**). By increasing the forward optic flow set point ω_{setFwd} at a given sideways optic flow set point $\omega_{setSide}$, one can change the robot's forward speed. By reducing the sideways optic flow set point at a given forward optic flow set point, one can induce a graceful shift from "wall-following behavior" to "centering behavior" [96]. "Centering behavior" occurs as a particular case of "wall-following behavior," whenever $\omega_{setSide} \leq \omega_{setFwd}/2$ [96]. In addition, the dual optic flow regulator requires a third feedback loop to stabilize the robot around its vertical axis, which makes the robot experience purely

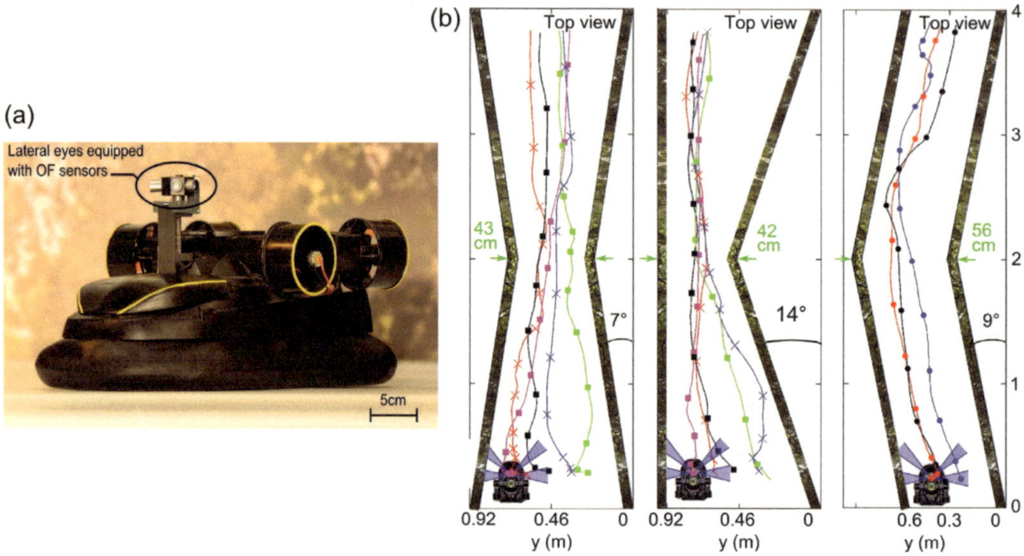

Figure 7. (a) A fully autonomous sighted hovercraft equipped with a minimalistic (8 pixel) compound eye. (b) Automatic wall-following behavior as the function of the initial ordinate in both tapered and bent corridors. (from [25] under CC-BY license).

translational optic flow. The robot's heading is maintained by a heading-lock system (based on a micro-compass enhanced by a micro-gyrometer) controlling the rear thrusters differentially in closed-loop mode (**Figure 6a**).

3.1.3. Bioinspired visuomotor convergence

Humbert put forward the bioinspired visuomotor convergence concept during his PhD degree (PhD thesis [100], obstacle avoidance and speed control [101, 102], terrain-following [103], corridor-following [92, 93, 104], urban canyon-following [105]) to control both land-based and flying robots solely on the basis of optic flow. This theory is based on the spatial decompositions performed by the neurons in the insect visuomotor system [106–108] that extract relative velocity and proximity information from patterns of optic flow. Advantages of bioinspired visuomotor convergence include:

- Significant improvements in signal-to-noise ratio of relative velocity and proximity information since one feedback signal is given across many estimates of optic flow [105].
- Through proper choice of weighting functions, the rotational and translational components can be separated automatically and do not require any derotation procedure [93].

To compare the bioinspired visuomotor convergence theory to the "optic flow balance strategy" that frequently fails in one-sided corridors or those with openings in a wall (see review [99]) or the switching mode strategy employed in such environments [87, 88], the bioinspired visuomotor convergence in [109, 110] retains the strategy of balancing lateral optic flows and leverages the stability and performance guarantees of the closed loop to achieve stable quadrotor flight in corridor-like environments which include large openings in a wall or additional structures such as small poles.

3.1.4. *Image expansion to avoid frontal obstacles*

The "optic flow balance strategy" was originally suggested to explain the centering behavior along a straight corridor (see review [99]). However, it turned out that this strategy, when used alone, did not allow an agent to avoid frontal obstacles, i.e., following a corridor that included L-junctions or T-junctions without using the frontal view field [111]. The frontal image expansion can therefore be used to estimate the time to contact [112] by means of the optic flow divergence [113, 114] and trigger a prespecified rotation angle around the robot's vertical axis. A simulated small helicopter could therefore trigger U-turns when encountering frontal obstacles [115], a wheeled robot could trigger a rotating angle of 90° [111] or of 110° [90] in front of an obstacle, or the robot could stop and rotate on the spot until the frontal range once again became large enough [88]. Other robots use a series of open-loop commands, called body saccades, to avoid a frontal obstacle. The saccade duration has either been set to a constant prespecified value [116, 117], determined according to a Gaussian distribution [118], or modulated using optic flow [119–123]. Recently, an optic flow-based algorithm has been developed to compute a quantified saccade angle; this has allowed a simulated fully actuated hovercraft to negotiate tight bends by triggering body saccades, on the basis of a time-to-contact criterion, and to realign its trajectory parallel to the wall along a corridor that includes sharp turns [124].

3.2. Obstacle avoidance in the vertical plane

Ventral optic flow can be used by aerial robots [125–127] to achieve different maneuvers: takeoff, terrain-following, flying nap of the earth, landing, and decking in the same way as honeybees do it [5, 97]. Ventral optic flow was also employed for ground avoidance onboard MAVs by maintaining the ventral optic flow at a given set point using a ventral optic flow regulator [95]. Another control algorithm based on a "bang-bang" method was used onboard MAVs to control their lift such that if a certain threshold of ventral optic flow was exceeded, the MAV elevator angle would be moved to a preset deflection [120, 121, 128].

Recently, the dual optic flow regulation principle applied in the vertical plane was tested onboard an 80-gram rotorcraft called BeeRotor [11]. As a third control feedback loop, an active system of reorientation based on a quasi-panoramic eye constantly realigned its gaze parallel to the nearest surface followed: BeeRotor demonstrated its abilities and achieved automatic terrain-following despite steep reliefs (**Figure 8**) without a need for inertial frames to access the verticality as flying insects do. Indeed, behavioral experiments performed 35 years ago on flying insects in zero gravity [129] or recent behavioral experiments with hymenopterans [37] or dipterans [130] demonstrated that flying insects do not actually sense verticality in flight by means of gravity perception as vertebrates do. The eye reorientation therefore enables BeeRotor, at an earlier stage, to detect the increase in the optic flow due to steep relief in order to properly avoid the obstacle [11]. Additionally, in the framework of the "Green Brain" project managed by James Marshall, a dual optic flow regulator for both speed control and lateral

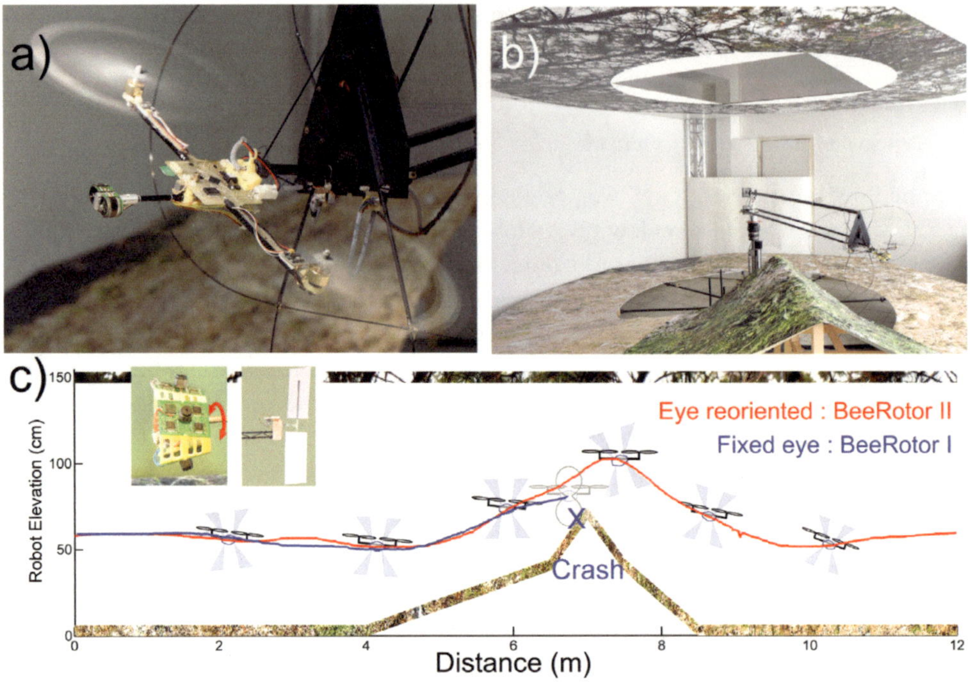

Figure 8. (a) BeeRotor I robot equipped with a twin CurvACE sensor [58]. (b) Experimental setup. (c) Trajectories of the robot BeeRotor II following the ground thanks to a dual optic flow regulator applied in the vertical plane and a fixed eye (blue traj.) or a decoupled eye (red traj.) oriented parallel to the ground (adapted from [11] under CC-BY license).

positioning and a ventral optic flow for altitude control were implemented onboard a small quadrotor [131].

3.3. Obstacle avoidance inside a maze

In silico experiments in a maze were mainly carried out in urban-like environments with a flying robot at a relatively high speed V_f in relatively wide urban canyons ([115] with V_f = 1 m/s and a minimum urban canyon width D_{min} = 4 m; [43] with V_f = 13 m/s and D_{min} = 40 m; [44] with V_f = 14 m/s and D_{min} = 50 m; [132] with V_f = 2 m/s and D_{min} = 10 m), hence generating an optic flow, coming from the walls, lower than 45°/s. On the other hand, navigating inside a building requires measuring not only the optic flow with a high refresh rate (>10 Hz), but also high optic flow magnitude in the range of those shown in **Figure 3** (i.e., >100°/s). In order to achieve this, the LORA robot is driven by a body saccadic system (see section 3.1.) and a dual optic flow regulator-based intersaccadic system (see section 3.1.) as depicted in detail in [124]. In **Figure 9**, the optic flow set points have been set at $\omega_{setSide} = 90^{\circ}/s$ and $\omega_{setFwd} = 130^{\circ}/s$; the LORA robot is seen to explore at $V_f = 0.33 \pm 0.21$ m/s inside the building and to adopt two possible routes along straight sections (following either the right wall or the left wall) according to Eqs. (9) and (10) leading to an operating point $V_{f\infty}$ = 0.48 m/s and y_{∞} = 0.31 m in a steady state. Except three lateral contacts with the walls (red crosses in **Figure 9**) where there are either a salient angle (90°) or a returning angle (270°), the LORA robot is able to explore for ~23 minutes inside the building even though it is fitted with a minimalistic visual system (16 pixel forming eight LMSs).

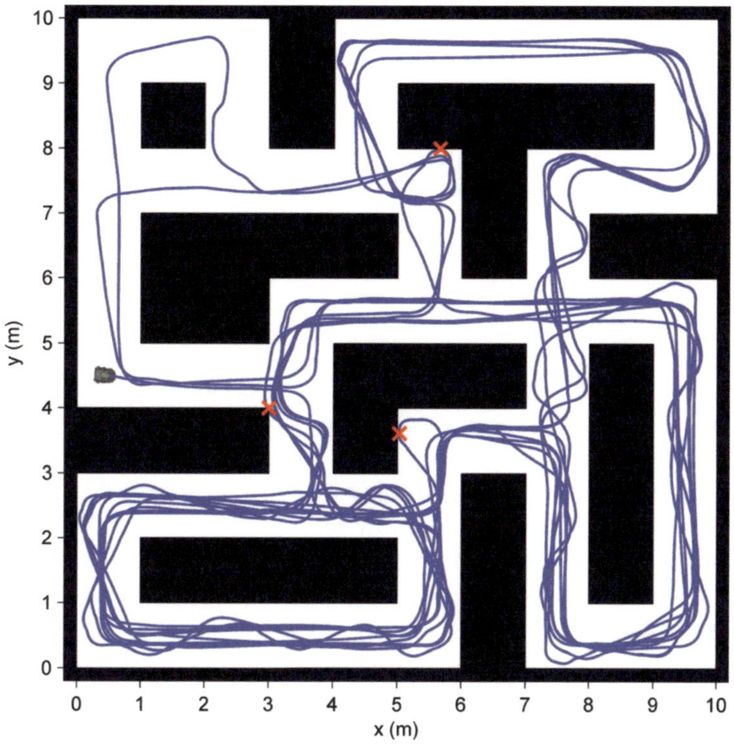

Figure 9. Trajectory of the LORA robot fitted with eight local motion sensors looking ahead at ±15°, ±30°, ±45°, and ±90° but also a heading-lock system by means of both a rate gyro and a micro compass. The LORA robot is driven by a body saccadic system (merging two incidence angles computed by ±30° and ±45° LMSs with Eq. (14) in [124]) and a dual optic flow regulator-based intersaccadic system as depicted in detail in [124]. This maze could represent corridors inside a building. The LORA robot starts at an initial position (X_0 = 0.5 m, Y_0=4.5 m) and with the initial heading $\Psi_0 = -5^{\circ}$ and progresses through the corridors including challenging junctions for ~23 minutes with only three lateral contacts with the walls (red crosses).

4. Drones in the field of architecture

Over the last decade, camera-equipped unmanned aerial vehicles (UAVs) are increasingly used in the field of architecture for visually monitoring construction, operation of buildings, and control of a failure of superstructures (skyscraper, stadium, chimney, nuclear area activity, bridges, etc.) [133]. UAVs can frequently survey construction sites, monitor work in progress, create documents for safety, and inspect existing structures, particularly for hard-to-reach areas. UAVs are used not only for 3D modeling for building reconstruction but also photogrammetric applications [134]. These UAVs evaluate their pose (i.e., their position and their orientation) in outdoor flight with a GPS giving an output signal of about 7 Hz (see section 1.3.) forcing drones to work away from structures, which is a drawback to take high-resolution pictures. In indoor flight, drones work in GPS-denied environments. Consequently, the use of active proximity sensors such as ultrasonic, laser range finders, radar, or scanning light detection and ranging (LIDAR) has been most of the time considered for this purpose [135]. However, such active sensors are bulky, high power consumption, low bandwidth, and low-output refresh rate (2 Hz–5 Hz), compromising their utility for UAV's fast maneuvers close to obstacles or walls. Recently, a lightweight sensor composed of four stereo heads and an inertial measurement unit (IMU) were developed to perform FPGA-based dense reconstruction for obstacle detection in all directions at 7 Hz output refresh rate [136]. In another application, a drone of a mass less than 500 g was developed for photogrammetric 3D reconstruction applied to a cultural heritage object [137] but requiring a motion capture system to determine accurately their pose of the robot at a frequency of 500 Hz. Better understanding how flying insects work will therefore help future drones to operate inside buildings where obstacles are very close.

5. Conclusion

The expanding set of roles for flying robots increasingly calls for them to operate at relatively high speed close to obstacles (<1 m) in all directions in GPS-denied or cluttered environments including buildings, warehouses, performance halls, or urban canyons. Tiny flying robots cannot rely on GPS signals in such complex environments. However, they have to pick up the 3D structure of the surrounding environment in real time to avoid collisions. At a short distance from obstacles (<1 m), the environment is completely unpredictable; most of the time, emissive proximity sensors have been considered for this purpose, but now optic flow sensing is truly becoming a part of MAV avionics in several companies (e.g., senseFly in Switzerland, Qualcomm or Centeye in the USA), and it can also be used as a direct feedback signal in MAV automatic guidance in the same way as flying insects use it.

Acknowledgements

The author wishes to thank N. Franceschini, S. Viollet, T. Raharijaona, and F. Ruffier for their fruitful discussions and to thank David Wood (English at your Service, www.eays.eu) for revising the English of the manuscript.

Author details

Julien R. Serres

Address all correspondence to: julien.serres@univ-amu.fr

Aix Marseille University, CNRS, ISM, Marseille, France

References

[1] Von Frisch K. The Dance Language and Orientation of Bees. Cambridge, Massachusetts: Harvard University Press; 1967

[2] Menzel R, Giurfa M. Cognitive architecture of a mini-brain: The honeybee. Trends in Cognitive Sciences. 2001;**5**(2):62-71

[3] Haddad D, Schaupp F, Brandt R, Manz G, Menzel R, Haase ANMR. Imaging of the honeybee brain. Journal of Insect Science. 2004;**4**(1):7

[4] Seidl R, Kaiser W. Visual field size, binocular domain and the ommatidial array of the compound eyes in worker honey bees. Journal of Comparative Physiology. 1981;**143**(1): 17-26

[5] Srinivasan MV, Zhang S, Altwein M, Tautz J. Honeybee navigation: Nature and calibration of the "odometer". Science. 2000;**287**(5454):851-853

[6] Srinivasan MV. Going with the flow: A brief history of the study of the honeybee's navigational 'odometer'. Journal of Comparative Physiology A. 2014;**200**(6):563-573

[7] Kv F. Gelöste und ungelöste Rätsel der Bienensprache. Die Naturwissenschaften. 1948; **35**(1):12-23

[8] von Helversen O, Edrich W. Der polarisationsempfänger im Bienenauge: ein Ultraviolettrezeptor. Journal of Comparative Physiology. 1974;**94**(1):33-47

[9] Ogawa Y, Ribi W, Zeil J, Hemmi JM. Regional differences in the preferred e-vector orientation of honeybee ocellar photoreceptors. Journal of Experimental Biology. 2017

[10] Landgraf T, Oertel M, Rhiel D, Rojas R. A biomimetic honeybee robot for the analysis of the honeybee dance communication system. IROS. 2010:3097-3102

[11] Expert F, Ruffier F. Flying over uneven moving terrain based on optic-flow cues without any need for reference frames or accelerometers. Bioinspiration & Biomimetics. 2015;**10**(2): 026003

[12] Webb B, Wystrach A. Neural mechanisms of insect navigation. Current Opinion in Insect Science. 2016;**15**:27-39

[13] Franz MO, Mallot HA. Biomimetic robot navigation. Robotics and Autonomous Systems. 2000;**30**:133-153

[14] Webb B. Can robots make good models of biological behaviour? Behavioral and Brain Sciences. 2001;**24**(06):1033-1050

[15] Webb B. Validating biorobotic models. Journal of Neural Engineering. 2006;**3**(3):R25

[16] Srinivasan MV. Visual control of navigation in insects and its relevance for robotics. Current Opinion in Neurobiology. 2011;**21**(4):535-543

[17] Floreano D, Ijspeert AJ, Schaal S. Robotics and neuroscience. Current Biology. 2014; **24**(18):R910-R920

[18] Ijspeert AJ. Biorobotics: Using robots to emulate and investigate agile locomotion. Science. 2014;**346**(6206):196-203

[19] Franceschini N. Small brains, smart machines: From fly vision to robot vision and back again. Proceedings of the IEEE. 2014;**102**(5):751-781

[20] Raharijaona T, Kerhuel L, Serres J, Roubieu F, Expert F, Viollet S, et al. Insect inspired visual motion sensing and flying robots. In: Handbook of Biomimetics and Bioinspiration: 2 Electromechanical Systems. World Scientific; 2014. pp. 565-611

[21] Franceschini N, Pichon JM, Blanes C. From insect vision to robot vision. Philosophical Transaction: Biological Sciences. 1992;**337**:283-294

[22] Franceschini N, Ruffier F, Serres J. A bio-inspired flying robot sheds light on insect piloting abilities. Current Biology. 2007;**17**(4):329-335

[23] Lambrinos D, Möller R, Labhart T, Pfeifer R, Wehner R. A mobile robot employing insect strategies for navigation. Robotics and Autonomous Systems. 2000;**30**(1):39-64

[24] Horchler AD, Reeve RE, Webb B, Quinn RD. Robot phonotaxis in the wild: A biologically inspired approach to outdoor sound localization. Advanced Robotics. 2004;**18**(8):801-816

[25] Roubieu FL, Serres JR, Colonnier F, Franceschini N, Viollet S, Ruffier F. A biomimetic vision-based hovercraft accounts for bees' complex behaviour in various corridors. Bioinspiration & Biomimetics. 2014;**9**(3):036003

[26] Duhamel PEJ, Pérez-Arancibia NO, Barrows GL, Wood RJ. Altitude feedback control of a flapping-wing microrobot using an on-board biologically inspired optical flow sensor. In: Robotics and Automation (ICRA), 2012 IEEE International Conference on. IEEE; 2012. p. 4228-4235

[27] Kushleyev A, Mellinger D, Powers C, Kumar V. Towards a swarm of agile micro quadrotors. Autonomous Robots. 2013;**35**(4):287-300

[28] Ma KY, Chirarattananon P, Fuller SB, Wood RJ. Controlled flight of a biologically inspired, insect-scale robot. Science. 2013;**340**(6132):603-607

[29] Dunkley O, Engel J, Sturm J, Cremers D. Visual-inertial navigation for a camera-equipped 25g nano-quadrotor. In: IROS2014 aerial open source robotics workshop; 2014

[30] Moore RJ, Dantu K, Barrows GL, Nagpal R. Autonomous MAV Guidance with a lightweight omnidirectional vision sensor. In: 2014 IEEE International Conference on Robotics and Automation (ICRA). IEEE; 2014. p. 3856-3861

[31] Floreano D, Wood RJ. Science, technology and the future of small autonomous drones. Nature. 2015;**521**(7553):460-466

[32] Gibson JJ. The Perception of the Visual World. Boston: Houghton Mifflin; 1950

[33] Whiteside TC, Samuel G. Blur zone. Nature. 1970;**225**:94-95

[34] Nakayama K, Loomis J. Optical velocity patterns, velocity-sensitive neurons, and space perception: A hypothesis. Perception. 1974;**3**(1):63-80

[35] Koenderink JJ, van Doorn AJ. Facts on optic flow. Biological Cybernetics. 1987;**56**(4):247-254

[36] Krapp HG, Hengstenberg R, et al. Estimation of self-motion by optic flow processing in single visual interneurons. Nature. 1996;**384**(6608):463-466

[37] Viollet S, Zeil J. Feed-forward and visual feedback control of head roll orientation in wasps (*Polistes humilis*, Vespidae, hymenoptera). Journal of Experimental Biology. 2013;**216**(7): 1280-1291

[38] Taylor GK, Krapp HG. Sensory systems and flight stability: What do insects measure and why? Advances in Insect Physiology. 2007;**34**:231-316

[39] Srinivasan M, Lehrer M, Kirchner W, Zhang S. Range perception through apparent image speed in freely flying honeybees. Visual Neuroscience. 1991;**6**(05):519-535

[40] Baird E, Srinivasan MV, Zhang S, Cowling A. Visual control of flight speed in honeybees. Journal of Experimental Biology. 2005;**208**(20):3895-3905

[41] Ibbotson M. Evidence for velocity–tuned motion-sensitive descending neurons in the honeybee. Proceedings of the Royal Society of London B: Biological Sciences. 2001; **268**(1482):2195-2201

[42] van der Zwaan S, Santos-Victor J. An insect inspired visual sensor for the autonomous navigation of a mobile robot. Proc of the Seventh International Sysposium on Intelligent Robotic Systems (SIRS). 1999

[43] Griffiths S, Saunders J, Curtis A, Barber B, McLain T, Beard R. Obstacle and terrain avoidance for miniature aerial vehicles. Advances in Unmanned Aerial Vehicles. Springer. 2007:213-244

[44] Beyeler A, Zufferey JC, Floreano D. Vision-based control of near-obstacle flight. Autonomous Robots. 2009;**27**(3):201-219

[45] Honegger D, Meier L, Tanskanen P, Pollefeys M. An open source and open hardware embedded metric optical flow cmos camera for indoor and outdoor applications. In: Robotics and Automation (ICRA), 2013 IEEE International Conference on. IEEE; 2013. pp. 1736-1741

[46] Burkhardt D, Gewecke M. Mechanoreception in Arthropoda: The chain from stimulus to behavioral pattern. In: Cold Spring Harbor symposia on quantitative biology. vol. 30. Cold Spring Harbor Laboratory Press; 1965. pp. 601-614

[47] Srinivasan MV. In: Wallman J, editor. How Insects Infer Range from Visual Motion. Miles FA: Elsevier Science Ltd; 1993

[48] Portelli G, Serres J, Ruffier F, Franceschini N. Modelling honeybee visual guidance in a 3-D environment. Journal of Physiology-Paris. 2010;**104**(1):27-39

[49] Portelli G, Ruffier F, Roubieu FL, Franceschini N. Honeybees' speed depends on dorsal as well as lateral, ventral and frontal optic flows. PLoS One. 2011;**6**(5):e19486

[50] Carroll D, Bidwell N, Laughlin S, Warrant E. Insect motion detectors matched to visual ecology. Nature. 1996;**382**(6586):63

[51] Franceschini N, Riehle A, Le Nestour A. Directionally selective motion detection by insect neurons. Facets of Vision. Springer. 1989:360-390

[52] Land MF. Visual acuity in insects. Annual Review of Entomology. 1997;**42**(1):147-177

[53] Rossel S. Regional differences in photoreceptor performance in the eye of the praying mantis. Journal of Comparative Physiology. 1979;**131**(2):95-112

[54] Land M. Optics and Vision in Invertebrates. In: Autrum H. Berlin Heidelberg New York: Springer; 1981

[55] Götz KG. Optomotorische untersuchung des visuellen systems einiger augenmutanten der fruchtfliege Drosophila. Kybernetik. 1964;**2**(2):77-92

[56] Horridge GA. The compound eye of insects. Scientific American. 1977;**237**:108-120

[57] Laughlin S, Weckström M. Fast and slow photoreceptors—A comparative study of the functional diversity of coding and conductances in the Diptera. Journal of Comparative Physiology A. 1993;**172**(5):593-609

[58] Floreano D, Pericet-Camara R, Viollet S, Ruffier F, Brückner A, Leitel R, et al. Miniature curved artificial compound eyes. Proceedings of the National Academy of Sciences. 2013;**110**(23):9267-9272

[59] Song YM, Xie Y, Malyarchuk V, Xiao J, Jung I, Choi KJ, et al. Digital cameras with designs inspired by the arthropod eye. Nature. 2013;**497**(7447):95-99

[60] Blanes C. Appareil visuel élémentaire pour la navigation à vue d'un robot mobile autonome. DEA thesis (Neurosciences), Univ Aix- Marseille. 1986

[61] Blanes C. Guidage visuel d'un robot mobile autonome d'inspiration bionique. PhD thesis, Institut National Polytechnique de Grenoble; 1991

[62] Franceschini N. Early processing of colour and motion in a mosaic visual system. Neuroscience Research Supplements. 1985;**2**:S17-S49

[63] Roubieu FL, Expert F, Boyron M, Fuschlock BJ, Viollet S, Ruffier F. A novel 1-gram insect based device measuring visual motion along 5 optical directions. In: Sensors, 2011 IEEE. IEEE. 2011. pp. 687-690

[64] Ruffier F, Viollet S, Amic S, Franceschini N. Bio-inspired optical flow circuits for the visual guidance of micro air vehicles. In: Circuits and Systems, 2003. ISCAS'03. Proceedings of the 2003 International Symposium on. vol. 3. IEEE; 2003. p. III-846

[65] Mafrica S, Godiot S, Menouni M, Boyron M, Expert F, Juston R, et al. A bio-inspired analog silicon retina with Michaelis-Menten auto-adaptive pixels sensitive to small and large changes in light. Optics Express. 2015;**23**(5):5614-5635

[66] Normann RA, Perlman I. The effects of background illumination on the photoresponses of red and green cones. The Journal of Physiology. 1979;**286**:491

[67] Matic T, Laughlin S. Changes in the intensity-response function of an insect's photoreceptors due to light adaptation. Journal of Comparative Physiology A: Neuroethology, Sensory, Neural, and Behavioral Physiology. 1981;**145**(2):169-177

[68] Laughlin S. The roles of parallel channels in early visual processing by the arthropod compound eye. Photoreception and Vision in Invertebrates. Springer. 1984:457-481

[69] Laughlin SB. Coding efficiency and design in visual processing. Facets of Vision. Springer. 1989:213-234

[70] Juusola M, French AS. Visual acuity for moving objects in first-and second-order neurons of the fly compound eye. Journal of Neurophysiology. 1997;**77**(3):1487-1495

[71] Riehle A, Franceschini N. Motion detection in flies: Parametric control over ON-OFF pathways. Experimental Brain Research. 1984;**54**(2):390-394

[72] Harris R, O'Carroll D. Afterimages in fly motion vision. Vision Research. 2002;**42**(14):1701-1714

[73] Hassenstein B, Reichardt W. Systemtheoretische analyse der zeit-, reihenfolgen-und vorzeichenauswertung bei der bewegungsperzeption des rüsselkäfers chlorophanus. Zeitschrift für Naturforschung B. 1956;**11**(9–10):513-524

[74] Reichardt W. Autocorrelation, a principle for the evaluation of sensory information by the central nervous system. Sensory Communication. 1961:303-317

[75] Kramer J, Sarpeshkar R, Koch C. An analog VLSI velocity sensor. In: Circuits and Systems, 1995. ISCAS'95, 1995 IEEE International Symposium on. vol. 1. IEEE; 1995. p. 413-416

[76] Moeckel R, Liu SC. Motion detection circuits for a time-to-travel algorithm. In: Circuits and Systems, 2007. ISCAS 2007. IEEE International Symposium on. IEEE. 2007. pp. 3079-3082

[77] Aubépart F, Franceschini N. Bio-inspired optic flow sensors based on FPGA: Application to micro-air-vehicles. Microprocessors and Microsystems. 2007;**31**(6):408-419

[78] Pudas M, Viollet S, Ruffier F, Kruusing A, Amic S, Leppävuori S, et al. A miniature bio-inspired optic flow sensor based on low temperature cofired ceramics (LTCC) technology. Sensors and Actuators A: Physical. 2007;**133**(1):88-95

[79] Expert F, Viollet S, Ruffier F. Outdoor field performances of insect-based visual motion sensors. Journal of Field Robotics. 2011;**28**(4):529-541

[80] Sabiron G, Chavent P, Raharijaona T, Fabiani P, Ruffier F. Low-speed optic-flow sensor onboard an unmanned helicopter flying outside over fields. Robotics and Automation (ICRA), 2013 IEEE International Conference on. IEEE. 2013:1742-1749

[81] Expert F, Roubieu FL, Ruffier F. Interpolation based "time of travel" scheme in a visual motion sensor using a small 2D retina. In: Sensors, 2012 IEEE. IEEE. 2012. pp. 1-4

[82] Mafrica S, Servel A, Ruffier F. Minimalistic optic flow sensors applied to indoor and outdoor visual guidance and odometry on a car-like robot. Bioinspiration & Biomimetics. 2016;**11**(6):066007

[83] Delbruck T, Mead CA. Adaptive photoreceptor with wide dynamic range. Circuits and Systems, 1994. ISCAS'94., 1994 IEEE International Symposium on. vol. 4. IEEE. 1994:339-342

[84] Xu P, Humbert JS, Abshire P. Analog VLSI implementation of wide-field integration methods. Journal of Intelligent & Robotic Systems. 2011;**64**(3–4):465-487

[85] Chao H, Gu Y, Napolitano M. A survey of optical flow techniques for robotics navigation applications. Journal of Intelligent & Robotic Systems. 2014;**73**(1–4):361

[86] Coombs D, Roberts K. Bee-bot: Using peripheral optical flow to avoid obstacles. In SPIE: Vol. 1825. Intelligent robots and computer vision XI. 1992:714-721

[87] Santos-Victor J, Sandini G, Curotto F, Garibaldi S. Divergent stereo in autonomous navigation: From bees to robots. International Journal of Computer Vision. 1995;**14**(2):159-177

[88] Weber K, Venkatesh S, Srinivasan MV. Insect inspired behaviors for the autonomous robots. In: Srinivasan MV, Venkatesh S, editors. From Living Eyes to Seeing Machines. 11. Oxford, UK: Oxford University Press; 1997. pp. 226-248

[89] Srinivasan MV, Chahl JS, Weber K, Venkatesh S, Nagle MG, Zhang SW. Robot navigation inspired by principles of insect vision. Robotics and Autonomous Systems. 1999; **26**(2):203-216

[90] Baratoff G, Toepfer C, Neumann H. Combined space-variant maps for optical flow navigation. Biological Cybernetics. 2000;**83**(3):199-209

[91] Argyros AA, Tsakiris DP, Groyer C. Biomimetic centering behavior for mobile robots with panoramic sensors. IEEE Robotics and Automation Magazine, Special issue on Mobile robots with panoramic sensors, Daniilides K, Papakolopoulos N, eds. 2004;**11**:21-30

[92] Humbert JS, Hyslop A, Chinn M. Experimental validation of wide-field integration methods for autonomous navigation. In: Intelligent Robots and Systems, 2007. IROS 2007. IEEE/RSJ International Conference on. San Diego, CA: IEEE; 2007. p. 2144-2149

[93] Humbert JS, Hyslop AM. Bioinspired visuomotor convergence. Robotics, IEEE Transactions on. 2010;**26**(1):121-130

[94] Roubieu FL, Serres J, Franceschini N, Ruffier F, Viollet S. A fully- autonomous hovercraft inspired by bees: wall following and speed control in straight and tapered corridors. In: Robotics and Biomimetics (ROBIO), 2012 IEEE International Conference on. IEEE; 2012. p. 1311-1318

[95] Ruffier F, Franceschini N. Optic flow regulation: The key to aircraft automatic guidance. Robotics and Autonomous Systems. 2005;**50**(4):177-194

[96] Serres J, Dray D, Ruffier F, Franceschini N. A vision-based autopilot for a miniature air vehicle: Joint speed control and lateral obstacle avoidance. Autonomous Robots. 2008; **25**(1–2):103-122

[97] Srinivasan M, Zhang S, Lehrer M, Collett T. Honeybee navigation en route to the goal: Visual flight control and odometry. The Journal of Experimental Biology. 1996;**199**(1):237-244

[98] Serres J, G M RF, Franceschini N. A bee in the corridor: Centering and wall-following. Die Naturwissenschaften. 2008;**95**:1181-1187

[99] Serres J, Ruffier F. Optic Flow-Based Robotics. In: Wiley Encyclopedia of Electrical and Electronics Engineering. John Wiley & Sons, Inc.; 2016. p. 1-14

[100] Humbert JS. Bio-inspired visuomotor convergence in navigation and flight control systems. California Institute of Technology; 2005

[101] Humbert JS, Murray RM, Dickinson MH. Sensorimotor convergence in visual navigation and flight control systems. In: Proceedings of the 16th IFAC World Congress. Praha, Czech Republic; 2005

[102] Humbert JS, Murray RM, Dickinson MH. A control-oriented analysis of bio-inspired visuomotor convergence. In: Decision and Control, 2005 and 2005 European Control Conference. CDC-ECC'05. 44th IEEE Conference on. IEEE; 2005. p. 245-250

[103] Humbert JS, Murray RM, Dickinson MH. Pitch-altitude control and terrain following based on bio-inspired visuomotor convergence. In: AIAA Conference on Guidance, Navigation and Control. vol. AIAA 2005–6280. San Francisco, CA; 2005

[104] Conroy J, Gremillion G, Ranganathan B, Humbert JS. Implementation of wide-field integration of optic flow for autonomous quadrotor navigation. Autonomous Robots. 2009;**27**(3):189-198

[105] Hyslop A, Krapp HG, Humbert JS. Control theoretic interpretation of directional motion preferences in optic flow processing interneurons. Biological Cybernetics. 2010;**103**(5): 353-364

[106] Hausen K. Motion sensitive interneurons in the optomotor system of the fly. Biological Cybernetics. 1982;**45**(2):143-156

[107] Krapp HG, Hengstenberg B, Hengstenberg R. Dendritic structure and receptive-field organization of optic flow processing interneurons in the fly. Journal of Neurophysiology. 1998;**79**(4):1902-1917

[108] Borst A, Haag J. Neural networks in the cockpit of the fly. Journal of Comparative Physiology A. 2002;**188**(6):419-437

[109] Keshavan J, Gremillion G, Escobar-Alvarez H, Humbert J. A analysis-based, controller-synthesis framework for robust bioinspired visual navigation in less-structured environments. Bioinspiration & Biomimetics. 2014;**9**(2):025011

[110] Keshavan J, Gremillion G, Alvarez-Escobar H, Humbert JS. Autonomous vision-based navigation of a Quadrotor in corridor-like environments. International Journal of Micro Air Vehicles. 2015;**7**(2):111-124

[111] Duchon AP, Warren WH. Robot navigation from a Gibsonian viewpoint. In: Systems, Man, and Cybernetics, 1994. Humans, Information and Technology., 1994 IEEE International Conference on. Vol. 3. IEEE. 1994. pp. 2272-2277

[112] Lee DNA. Theory of visual control of braking based on information about time-to-collision. Perception. 1976;**5**(4):437-459

[113] Nelson R, Aloimonos J. Using flow field divergence for obstacle avoidance in visual navigation. In: Science Applications International Corp, Proceedings: Image Understanding Workshop. vol. 2; 1988

[114] Ancona N, Poggio T. Optical Flow From 1D Correlation: Application to a Simple Time-To-Crash Detector. In: 4th International Conference on Computer Vision, Proceedings of the. Berlin, Germany; 1993. p. 209-214

[115] Muratet L, Doncieux S, Briere Y, Meyer JA. A contribution to vision- based autonomous helicopter flight in urban environments. Robotics and Autonomous Systems. 2005;**50**(4): 195-209

[116] i Badia SB, Bernardet U, Verschure PF. Non-linear neuronal responses as an emergent property of afferent networks: A case study of the locust lobula giant movement detector. PLoS Computational Biology. 2010;**6**(3):e1000701

[117] Zufferey JC, Floreano D. Fly-inspired visual steering of an ultralight indoor aircraft. IEEE Transactions on Robotics. 2006;**22**(1):137-146

[118] Reiser MB, Dickinson MH. A test bed for insect-inspired robotic control. Philosophical Transactions of the Royal Society of London A: Mathematical, Physical and Engineering Sciences. 2003;**361**(1811):2267-2285

[119] Beyeler A, Zufferey JC, Floreano D. 3D vision-based navigation for indoor microflyers. In: Robotics and Automation, 2007 IEEE International Conference on. IEEE; 2007. p. 1336-1341

[120] Barrows GL, Neely C, Miller KT. Optic flow sensors for MAV navigation. In: Fixed and Flapping Wing Aerodynamics for Micro Air Vehicle Applications. Bellingham, U.S.A.: Progress in Astronautics and Aeronautics, AIAA, Vol. 195. 2001. pp. 557-574

[121] Green WE, Oh PY, Barrows G. Flying insect inspired vision for autonomous aerial robot maneuvers in near-earth environments. In: Robotics and Automation, 2004. Proceedings. ICRA'04. 2004 IEEE International Conference on. vol. 3. IEEE; 2004. p. 2347-2352

[122] Lindemann JP, Weiss H, Möller R, Egelhaaf M. Saccadic flight strategy facilitates collision avoidance: Closed-loop performance of a cyberfly. Biological cybernetics. 2008;**98**(3): 213-227

[123] Rezaei M, Saghafi F. Optical flow-based obstacle avoidance of a fixed-wing MAV. Aircraft Engineering and Aerospace Technology. 2011;**83**(2):85-93

[124] Serres JR, Ruffier F. Biomimetic autopilot based on minimalistic motion vision for navigating along corridors comprising U-shaped and S-shaped turns. Journal of Bionic Engineering. 2015;**12**(1):47-60

[125] Chahl JS, Srinivasan MV, Zhang SW. Landing strategies in honeybees and applications to uninhabited airborne vehicles. International Journal of Robotics Research. 2004;**23**(2): 101-110

[126] Garratt MA, Chahl JS. Vision-based terrain following for an unmanned rotorcraft. Journal of Field Robotics. 2008;**25**(4–5):284-301

[127] Herissé B, Hamel T, Mahony R, Russotto FX. Landing a VTOL unmanned aerial vehicle on a moving platform using optical flow. IEEE Transactions on Robotics. 2012;**28**(1):77-89

[128] Green WE, Oh PY. Optic-flow-based collision avoidance. IEEE Robotics & Automation Magazine. 2008;**15**(1)

[129] Nelson TE, Peterson JR. NSTA-NASA Shuttle Student Involvement Project. Experiment Results: Insect Flight Observation at Zero Gravity. 1982

[130] Goulard R, Vercher JL, Viollet S. To crash or not to crash: How do hoverflies cope with free-fall situations and weightlessness? Journal of Experimental Biology. 2016;**219**(16): 2497-2503

[131] Sabo C, Cope A, Gurny K, Vasilaki E, Marshall JA. Bio-inspired visual navigation for a Quadcopter using optic flow. In: AIAA Infotech @ Aerospace; 2016. p. 0404

[132] Garratt MA, Cheung A. Obstacle Avoidance in Cluttered Environments Using Optic Flow. In: Australian Conference on Robotics and Automation; 2009

[133] Ham Y, Han KK, Lin JJ, Golparvar-Fard M. Visual monitoring of civil infrastructure systems via camera-equipped Unmanned Aerial Vehicles (UAVs): a review of related works. Visualization in Engineering. 2016;**4**(1):1

[134] Küng O, Strecha C, Fua P, Gurdan D, Achtelik M, Doth KM, et al. Simplified building models extraction from ultra-light UAV imagery. ISPRS-international archives of the photogrammetry. Remote Sensing and Spatial Information Sciences. 2011;**3822**:217-222

[135] Holz D, Nieuwenhuisen M, Droeschel D, Schreiber M, Behnke S. Towards multimodal omnidirectional obstacle detection for autonomous unmanned aerial vehicles. Int Arch Photogramm Remote Sens Spatial Inf Sci(ISPRS). 2013;**1**:W2

[136] Gohl P, Honegger D, Omari S, Achtelik M, Pollefeys M, Siegwart R. Omnidirectional visual obstacle detection using embedded FPGA. In: Intelligent robots and systems (IROS), 2015 IEEE/RSJ International conference on. IEEE; 2015. p. 3938-3943

[137] Louiset T, Pamart A, Gattet E, Raharijaona T, De Luca L, Ruffier F. A shape-adjusted tridimensional reconstruction of cultural heritage artifacts using a miniature Quadrotor. Remote Sensing. 2016;**8**(10):858

Chapter 4

Biomimetic Design for a Bioengineered World

Irem Deniz and Tugba Keskin-Gundogdu

Additional information is available at the end of the chapter

http://dx.doi.org/10.5772/intechopen.72912

Abstract

Biodesign can be explained as a method that includes various researches and applications related to taking inspiration from natural functions, systems, components, or processes in solving a problem. Accordingly, biodesign is commonly used in the design of artificial devices, structures, and buildings in the field of bioengineering. The recent developments in the field of biotechnology and bioengineering bring out various products that are designed in collaboration with different engineering disciplines. In this chapter, the possible use of bacteria, microalgae, and fungi for biomimetic design and the role of biomimicry for these designs will be briefly discussed.

Keywords: bioengineering, biomimetic design, biodesign, microalgae, fungi, bacteria

1. Introduction

Biodesign, in which living organisms can be used as a design input, is a study field that takes nature as an example and aims to make sustainable, functional, durable, and nonhealth threatening products. In literature, biodesign appears together with concepts such as biomimetics, biomimicry, design inspired by nature and morphogenic design [1]. Bioengineering is the application of engineering's analytical, mathematical, and result-oriented approaches to the world of biology, while traditional engineering approaches focus on just mathematical and physical applications to solve the problems or produce a product; bioengineering uses all the information about life, human, and all living organisms. This area includes all the necessary sciences. Bioengineering deals not just with scientific knowledge but also with engineering approaches. In addition to this, biodesign is a methodological approach of new innovations inspired by nature or using the living organism itself to make life easier. The biodesign aims to be ecological, environmental friendly, and also economical. Bioengineering is a scientific discipline that fully encompasses the applications of biodesign [2].

Recently, researchers working in areas such as biology, engineering, architecture, and chemistry have come together to work on bioengineered design. The concept of bioengineered design must be absolutely interdisciplinary [3]. As is known, there are great differences between the language used by basic scientists and engineers. However, it is tried to find common points in these studies. With the accomplishment of this challenging task, a great new generation of biologically inspired design products emerges [4].

It is thought that the biologically inspired design process can take place in six steps. In the first step, the problem needs to be identified. At this point, there is a problem that has not been noticed before, or a solution that has been proposed before but considered inadequate, like reduction of water losses, more benefit from the sun, etc. The second step is to determine the boundaries of the problem. At this stage, the main objectives of reaching a solution point are determined by a biological solution that is sought in the third step. At this point, biologically based approaches that may be probing solutions are searched and possible solutions are identified. Accordingly, there will be some questions to be answered such as, Should a microorganism be used? Should living conditions of a living thing be imitated? In the fourth step, the biological solution is examined in detail. The information on this subject is compiled, and the outline of the work is settled, and the principles of the fifth step are determined. In the sixth step application, bioengineered material suitable for the target and purpose is realized [5].

An overview of biologically inspired design products emerging as the greatest indication that bioengineering and other sciences is harmoniously integrated into this chapter. The products and their areas of use emerged by the designers in this field were examined in general terms. Since our primary goal is to emphasize the importance of bioengineering approach in the field of biodesign and biomimicry, we have not mentioned the detailed metabolic pathways in the products and the issues discussed.

This chapter introduces the usage of microbiology, algal technology, fungal technology, and biomaterials into biomimicry and biodesign field. In each section, the approaches proposed by different researchers on the subject under the relevant heading and the resulting products are explained in detail. By the end of the chapter, the future prospects and potential applications of biomimetic design are discussed. Considering the recent trends across the globe, a full discussion of recent examples is included to raise the awareness of bioinspired and bioengineered materials.

2. Bacteria for biodesign

This section focuses on the role of bacteria in biodesign and biomimicry. The used biological processes with bacteria or using the properties of bacteria will be considered as important alternatives instead of industrial technologies. The given examples are related to direct bacterial production of some biodesign concepts or to use the biomimicry for a bacterial production or to model a bacterial behavior. In short terms, bacteria could take a very big role in biomimicry and biodesign and many of their abilities are waiting to be discovered.

http://dx.doi.org/10.5772/intechopen.72912

According to the United Nations reports [6], desertification will be one of the important environmental crises of future life. Currently, 100–200 million people are threatened by the hard living conditions of desert life. The most affected countries are Sudan, Chad, and Nigeria. One of the solutions of desertification could be microbial-induced calcium production. The process occurs by using the bacteria, urea, and calcium source to solidify the sand at 24 h. The role of an architect with this process is to choose the best place for the structure. Using the ability of sandstone production of some types of bacteria is the most studied subject of biodesign concept. An interesting concept for the conditions of a desert life was proposed by Magnus Larsson from Architectural Association, London. Sandstone formation in the desert can be turned into architectural building structures from sand in a desert to act as a barrier to be protected against spread of desert (**Figure 1**). The ability of *Bacillus pasteurii* can be used to harden the very small sand particles into a nonintended but organized architectural structure. The shape of this structure designed by nature will serve as a protector for tress, collector of moisture, and a shelter for thousands of people with a very low cost [7]. Also, Turkey Biodesign Team, an interactive and creative platform built by the academicians of bioengineering, architecture, electrical & electronics engineering, and civil engineering, had studied hardening sand for structural materials [8]. The main aim of their first study is to build a children's playground made by biocalcification of sand, which will be totally biological and nontoxic. The ability of microorganism to harden sand will be the main process of this project. The playground will have tunnel like holes and some areas to slip down. It will be an ecological and economical alternative for plastic-based playgrounds, which are generally used worldwide.

Another application of the cementation ability of *B. pasteurii* is Biobrick proposed by BIOMASON (**Figure 2**). The brick is the smallest part of a building, and it is known as the oldest construction component that has been used for thousands of years. It has a very simple form, and there is no need for specialized engineering skills, materials, or technologies for production [9]. However, these conventional basic and old technologies have some disadvantages in the view of environment such as intense energy consumption in terms of heat, high amount of toxic gas release during production, and the usage of agricultural soil. These factors cause a

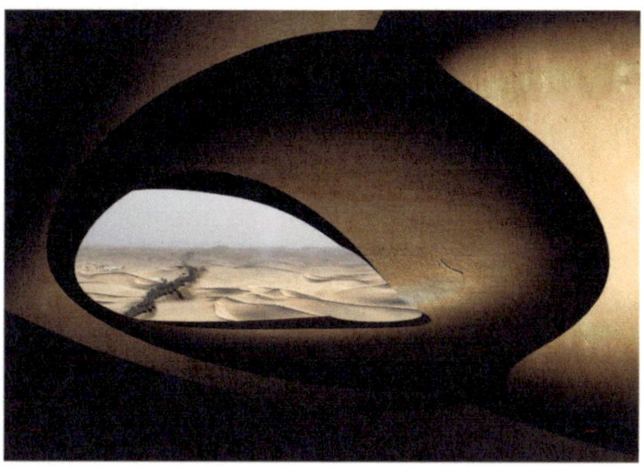

Figure 1. The schematic view of DUNE by Magnus LARSSON (taken from Flicker).

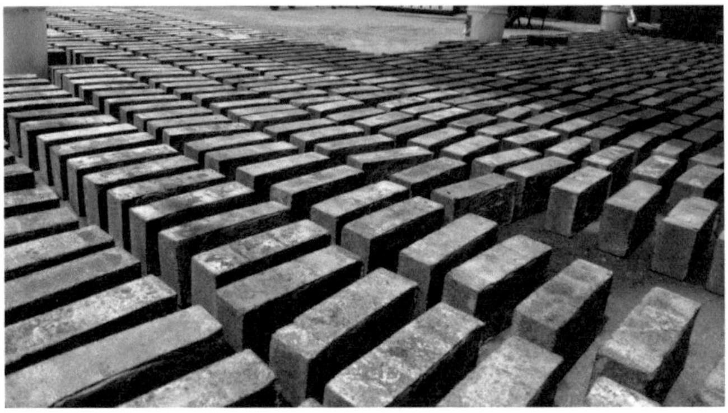

Figure 2. Biobrick that was built by Biomason.

very high-carbon footprint of brick formation industry. Biobrick uses the microbial cementation process by *B. pasteurii* to produce a rigid shape with high durability and strength similar to conventional bricks. The production times of Biobrick takes 3 days, which is the same as a conventional brick. Application of a comparison in terms of carbon footprint will be resulted in the superiority of Biobricks. In the view of environment and human health, Biobrick is the most ecofriendly solution for building industry [10].

The last application of the microbial cementation is to use their ability to produce $CaCO_3$ to heal the cracks of the buildings. The effect of nature such as wind, rain, and the temperature changes can be resulted in cracking of the conventional and also the biobricks. Application of a healing procedure will improve the durability and strength of the brick and also the lifetime of a building. Jonkers group in Delft University has a publication on the healing process of the cracks with different types of calcifying bacteria and the healing could be clearly seen from SEM shots clearly (**Figure 3**). Using a natural process for a building is the best environmental friendly and sustainable solution [11].

A sustainable world is the main focus of many researchers. The clean and renewable energy production is the first step of a sustainable environment and the world. The consumption of organic materials increased directly proportional to the population growth and the need of disposal of organic wastes is one of the main problems especially for developing countries. Bioenergy production is one of the important subjects of the sustainable environment, and the anaerobic digestion is the key step of bioenergy production. Anaerobic digestion is a biomimicry process. The ability of converting lignocellulosic biomass into methane by intestinal activity of herbivory animals is mimicked in an anaerobic digester for methane formation. About 200 billions of lignocellulosic biomass is produced, and considerable part of this biomass is disposed into environment without any treatment. The energy potential of these wastes can be used for bioenergy production in an anaerobic digester to improve the quality of life and a sustainable environment [12].

This biomimicry concept can be applied in a house for biodesign using these anaerobic bacteria. A microdigester can be designed to convert the food waste already released at home to supply the energy to cook the food, and the digestate from the anaerobic digester can

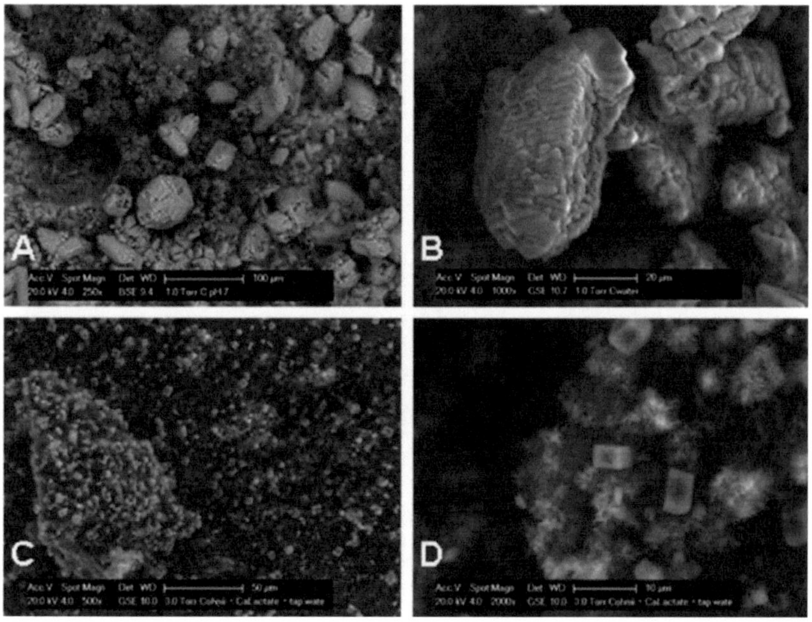

Figure 3. Self-healing cementation by Allain Jonkers. Cement stone specimens with incorporated healing agent (B. cohnii spores plus calcium lactate), cracked after 7 (panels A: 250× and B: 1000× magnification), or 28 days curing (panels C: 500× and D: 2000× magnification). The relatively large (20–80 μm sized) mineral precipitates visible on crack surfaces of young specimens (A and B) are presumably due to bacterial conversion of calcium lactate to calcium carbonate. The small (2–5 μm sized) precipitates on crack surfaces of older specimens (C and D), larger bacterial precipitates are not produced here likely due to loss of viability of cement stone embedded bacterial spores (taken from [2]).

be used as a fertilizer for the vegetable growth to increase the quality of soil and compost. Microbial Home concept is proposed by Jack Mama and Clive Van Heerden based on this idea (**Figure 4**). The components of the microbial digester work in a cyclic way that resembles an ecosystem of a house [13].

Cellulose and textile materials are known to be the main causes of environmental pollution. For the design of furnish of the house of any type of cover material bacterial cellulose and bacterial textile could be the biological and environmental friendly solutions [14]. Natural biopolymers produced by bacterial activity can also be used for medical applications [15]. Suzanne Lee used the microbial cellulose in her textile design (**Figure 5**). The microbial cellulose is combination of millions of bacteria grown in bathtubs of sweet green tee to produce clothing. Growing leather without an animal is one of the important applications of bacteria for biodesign.

The biomimicry of foraging strategy of the bacteria helps to find a way of optimization of bioprocess. The artificial potential field method in autonomous vehicle guidance has many similarities between foraging algorithms of a bacteria. The uninhabited autonomous vehicles generally used in military are optimized by an algorithm derived from the foraging behavior of *Escherichia coli*. The chemotaxis behavior of *E. coli* was used to derive the algorithm for these vehicles [16].

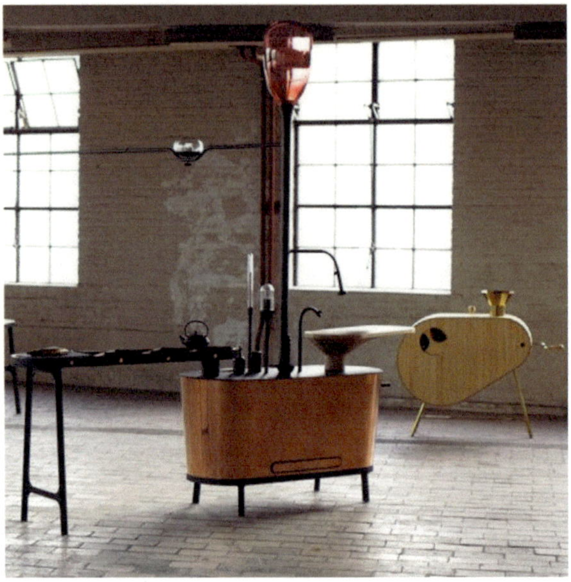

Figure 4. Microbial home by Philips Design (taken from deezen.com).

Biodesign and biomimicry is an emerging strategy to evolve the biological systems for application to create novel technologies for a sustainable world and environment. What types of products can be produced by bacteria? How bacteria reacts to a outer instigation? How their ability can be applied to bioprocess studies? There are a lot of questions waiting to be answered for biomimicry and biodesign world.

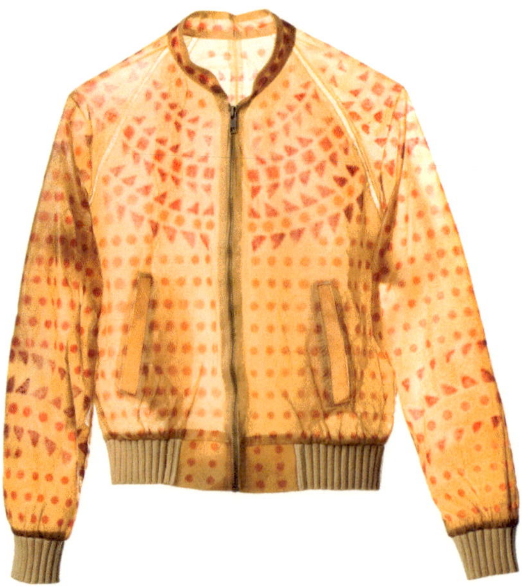

Figure 5. Biocouture by Suzanne Lee (taken from biocouture.com).

3. Microalgal technologies for biodesign

The field of biodesign has risen as a stimulating new multidisciplinary field that merges the inspirer solutions from nature with the cutting edge of modern technology, encouraging technological discoveries that could let people to live sustainable and economic lives, more in unity with the environment. Microalgae are considered as the one of the most attractive bio-based sources with its specific properties.

Microalgae are photosynthetic microorganisms and they generally are adapted to live in extreme conditions due to their unicellular or simple multicellular structure [17]. Microalgae exist in almost all ecosystems, both aquatic and terrestrial. It is considered that there are more than 50,000 strains; however, only half of them have been defined and studied.

Microalgae play a great role in the removal of the CO_2, which makes them sustainable and environmentally friendly. They use inorganic carbon and light energy to produce fuel for the microalgal activities. This functional property attracted the bioengineers and architectures attention to investigate their possible usage in constructive structures for a sustainable inhabiting. As an example, designer Adam Miklosi was inspired by the concept of mutualism to create a futuristic oxygen bar called the Chlorella Pavilion where exhausted people can relax and fill up their energy with the oxygen-rich air (**Figure 6**). Basically, Miklosi aimed to design a piping system where living microalgae can be introduced through the structure to create an algae fountain. Humans relaxing (and breathing) in this structure would give the microalgae the CO_2 it needs to survive, and in exchange, the microalgae (strain *Chlorella* sp.) would give the visitors an extra oxygen push-up [18].

The BIQ House in Hamburg was defined as the world's first microalgae-powered building in the world. The SSC (Strategic Science Consult of Germany), a bioreactor technology company, Arup (Concept Design) an international design consultant and Colt International, a reactor design company are the three partners who developed biofacade concept. This facade is an example of a 200-m^2 building as residence with an integrated concept of microalgal photobioreactors, and with this building, heat can be produced from this reactor. Other important properties of this house are dynamic shading, thermal insulation, and abatement of noise. The three partners are developing new projects for production of larger scale buildings with commercial benefits [19].

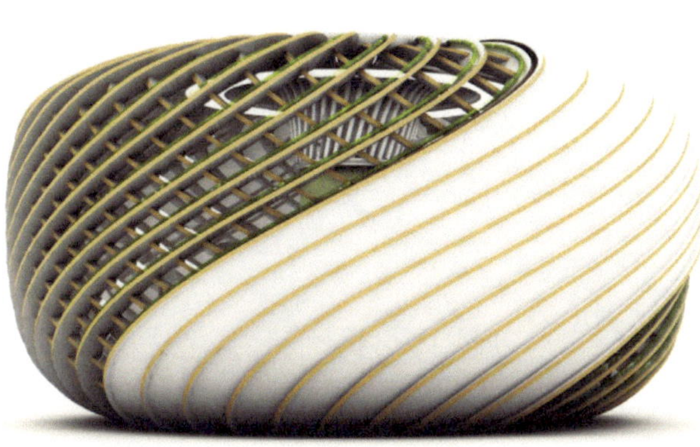

Figure 6. Chlorella Pavilion by Adam Miklosi (taken from inhabitat.com).

The Algaevator, designed by Jie Zhang and Tyler Stevermer, can be given as another project example [20]. This structure basically composed of an microalgae farm to be used as a transparent roofing system that can be used in neglected buildings to help regenerate urban environments and with that unique structure, the Algaevator can be considered as gravity-based photobioreactor (**Figure 7**). This microalgal-roof can be used for various purposes as important products and alternative fuels. This funnel-shaped structure also optimizes sun exposure for microalgae production and can also harvest rainwater for additional sustainability [20].

Environmental concerns on nonsustainability and petroleum-based source decrease are considered as the main issues that we currently face. Microalgae-integrated buildings serve a sustainable solution to these problems. Several architects and designers have used these microorganisms in their conceptual constructive structures. The microalgae facades have functional properties conducted to take advantageous of microalgae considering its property to decrease CO_2 emission. The breathing-light-responsive facade, which can open and close according to temperature changes, is a part of Abu Dhabi towers (**Figure 8**). When it is dark (night), the windows would still be closed, whereas in the day time, it would be opened to let the aeration of the building [21].

Microalgae is not only used for their property of absorbing CO_2 emissions but also for other purposes. In a project conducted by HOK in LA, the algae facade was designed to clean wastewater and to filter throughway supporting shading for interior area. It was also targeted to produce lipids that can be converted into biofuel [22]. Another cognitive project is Algae Urban Farm in Tehran, Iran proposed by ecoLogic Studio (**Figure 9**). The project also conducted as a photobioreactor tube supplies cooling strategies through its shading effect with natural ventilation. Besides, this microalgal facade plays a role as a heat regulator [23]. In addition to these projects, Battery Park project in San Francisco was carried out to reduce the net energy to zero while reducing CO_2 levels [24].

Microalgae also have applications for esthetic purposes in architectural structures that lead to an impressive design outcomes with its different geometric variations and characteristic colors. Also, microalgae-based facades provide sustainable productions in such areas where

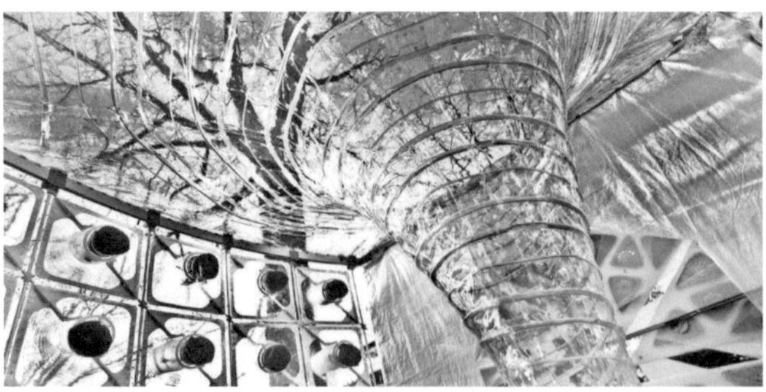

Figure 7. Algaevator (taken from domusweb.it).

http://dx.doi.org/10.5772/intechopen.72912

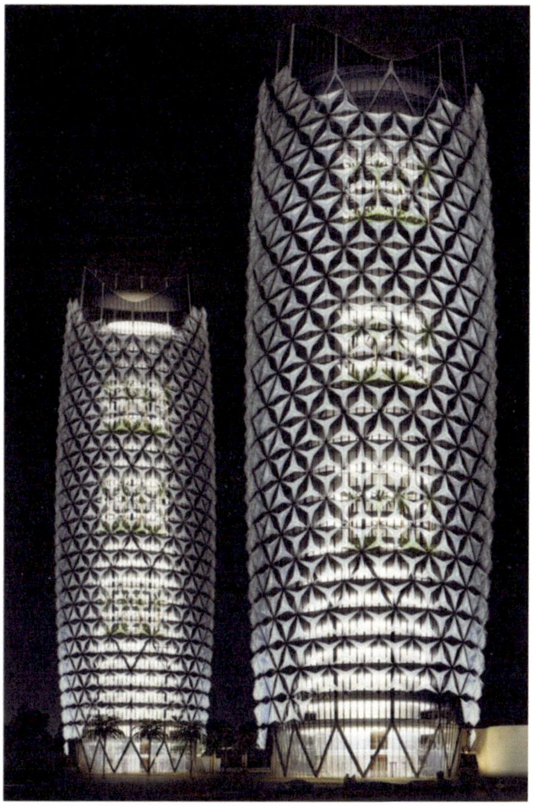

Figure 8. Abu Dhabi Towers (taken from ihabitat.com).

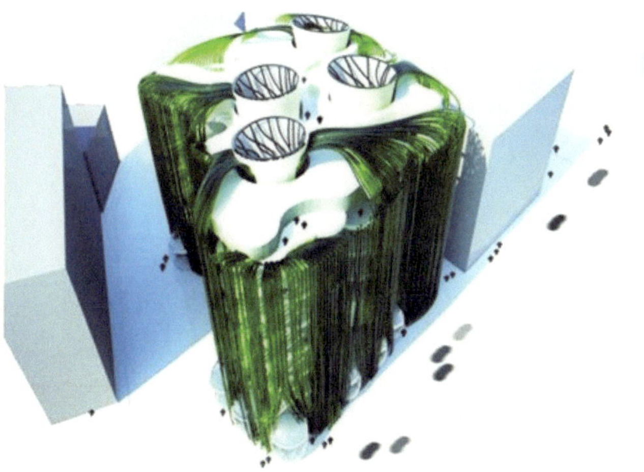

Figure 9. Algae Urban Farm in Tehran, Iran (taken from 33rdsquare.com).

no other structures can be built. The Biodesign Institute at Arizona State University was built, which is a new structure built in the desert called "tubes in desert" to produce energy engine fuel in a more sustainable way. The microalgae live in the tubes with enhanced light penetration to produce biofuel within an esthetic way [25].

4. Fungi for biodesign

Living organisms can provide a new approach for architectural structures. Bioengineers and architects are working on the research of biodegradable materials produced by microorganisms with novel functions. Fungus can also be considered as a biodesign material for durable and hard structures.

Fungi have approximately 100,000 known species, are eukaryotic, and belong to the kingdom *Fungi*, including molds, yeast, and mushrooms. Fungi are the most abundant organisms on Earth and have great applications for food and medical industry for centuries [26]. Recently, researchers used these organisms to build living structures for economic and environmental friendly designs. The living project, for example, is considered as one of the most comprehensive designs that was planned to build towers made from corn stalks and fungi (**Figure 10**). This structure is a product with a circular lifecycle in which fungi feeds using corn stalks. This tower first starts as fungus and plant matter, then transforms into bricks, finally biodegraded, and mixed into soil serving as fertilizers [27].

Moreover, fungi have the capability of being strong, water and fire resistant, and can be used as building materials. After drying, the mycelium can be used as a strong concrete material to obtain any kind of shape desired. From this point forth, designer Eric Klarenbeek in collaboration with researchers at the University of Wageningen produced 3D printed chairs out of mycelium (the vegetative part of a fungus) (**Figure 11**) that makes for a surprisingly solid, strong, lightweight, organic, compostable, and durable material for furniture [28].

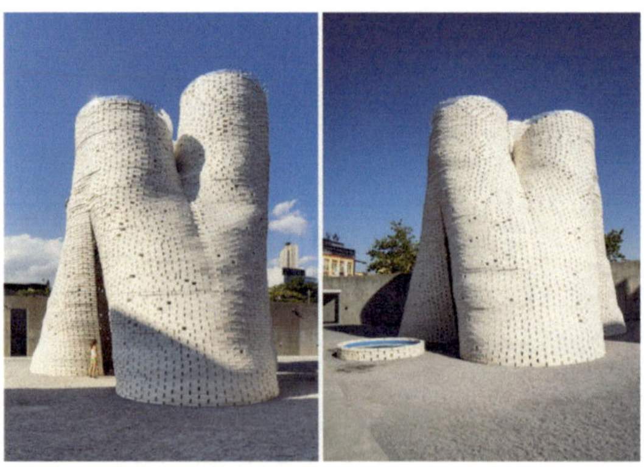

Figure 10. The living project (taken from designboom.com).

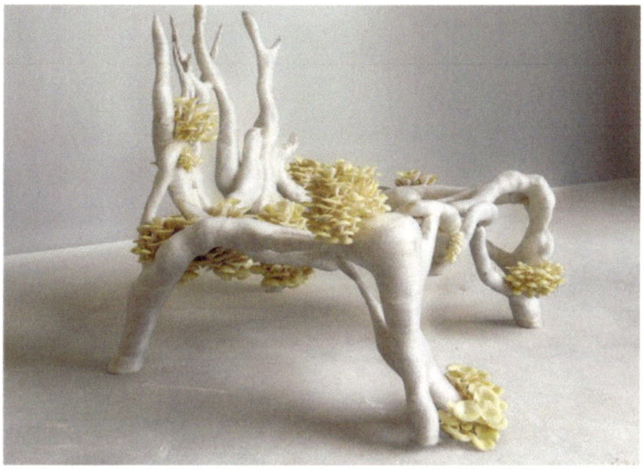

Figure 11. A fungus chair (taken from dezeen.com).

As another example for durable structures, a new small-scale company in Turkey, called Diploid Biotechnological Products, is working on a project to make an environmentally friendly insulation material out of fungi that is thinner and stronger than conventional substitutes [29].

Furthermore, New York-based nonprofits Terreform ONE and Genspace created Mycoform, a durable and 100% compostable material made from fungi, wood chips, gypsum, oat bran, and other biological materials (**Figure 12**). The mycoform production process is pollution-free, sustainable, and requires low energy. This material is produced by agricultural wastes and after inoculation with *Ganoderma lucidum* in a place with higher humidity, the fungi consumes the cellulose in the byproducts to create a branch-like network. Then, the branching mycelia grow rapidly into a weight-bearing structure [30]. Likewise, large-scale production examples for biodesign materials that use fungi are also available.

Ecovative Design in the United States commercially produce a packing material as a competitive alternative to petroleum polymer foam that represents 25% of waste landfill sites and contains toxins such as benzene. Their products are made from mycelium that is grown using local agricultural wastes and are uniquely rigid and dense [7]. As an another industrial application, Microbial Home Project developed by Philips in the Netherlands (**Figure 13**) provides various integrated appliances that refrigerate heat, generate food and help in treatment of wastes utilizing bacteria, fungi, and other naturally occurring organisms to mimic an ecosystem and to enable each natural process [7].

Slime molds and oomycetes (water molds) are fungus-like organisms, but they belong to kingdom *Chromista*; however, they are often called fungi, as well. Slime molds (*Physarum polycephalum*) are eukaryotic organisms that can grow as single cell or flocs in the dark. Unlike any other organisms, slime molds have discovered to have a unique intelligence and that they can learn and predict the laboratory conditions that are unfavorable [31]. Using those abilities, a group of researchers from Hokkaido University worked with the slime mold *P. polycephalum* in a humid plate, where they placed the mold in the central position of the plate of Tokyo map and

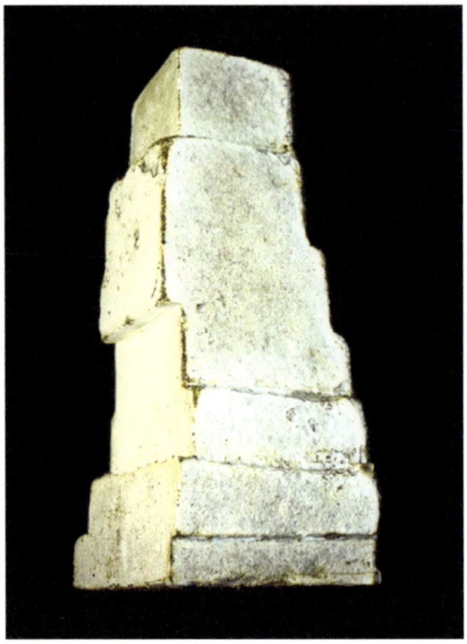

Figure 12. New Museum NYC grown of mycoform (taken from terreform.org).

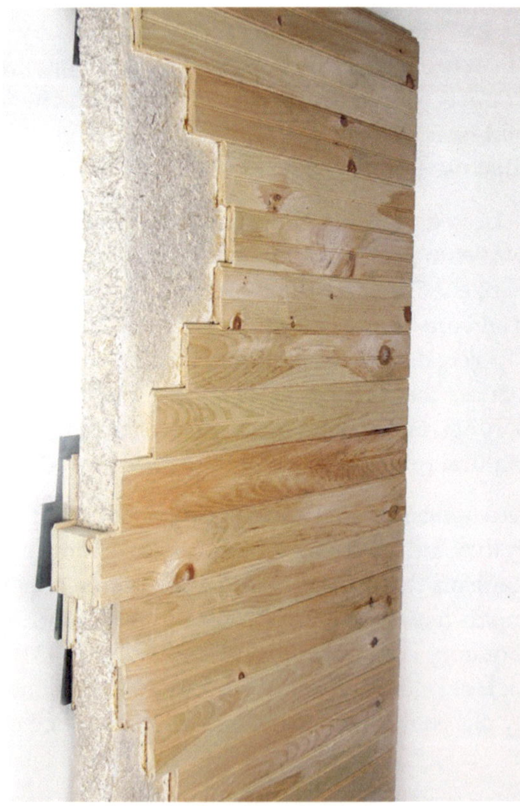

Figure 13. A sustainable design product (taken from dezeen.com).

again put oat flakes for feeding the mold on the major cities of Tokyo. In the plate, illuminating materials were used to mimic mountainous area and as *Physarum* avoids bright light, it grew and spread through the pathway of water and oats in the plate. Firstly, the mold was filled in the plate with plasmodia (its living single form cell) and then thinned by the network creating branches to utilize the nutrition efficiently. The final network uniquely and strikingly resembled Tokyo's rail system [32]. Till then, several studies are performed and reported to show the unambiguous potential of the strain. Such as, a similar approach for Izmir map has been conducted as a new project by Turkish Biodesign Team. The same strain will be used for designing the walking ways of a special area of Izmir, Turkey. Besides, the studies of the unconventional computing through the practice of architecture for slime molds are still in development.

5. Biomaterials for biodesign

Biomedical engineering is one of the most comprehensive fields of study of bioengineering. Improvement in patient's health, the development of new creative and painless surgical techniques, the fight with disability, and even the design and production of vital replacements can be done by biomedical applications [33].

A biomaterial is any concept that is in interaction with biological systems. This concept can be a matter, a surface, or an artificial tissue. They can be provided directly from nature or synthesized by new, innovative bioengineering approaches. Regenerative medicine and tissue engineering are the main areas that cover biomaterials. A lot of new organs or replacements of human body can be produced such as prosthesis veins and heart valves, etc. [34].

It is thought that the first biomaterial applications were made in Mayans time. Findings show that Mayan's use some shells in dental operations. In the following years, metals, such as silver, gold, and titanium, have been used in some parts of the body. In the following years, biomaterials that are compatible with body tissues have been studied [34].

Biomaterials must carry many important criteria in order to adapt to living life:

- Be very resistant to environmental conditions such as heat, pressure, and humidity.
- Have low friction coefficients (for use in joints).
- It must be multifunctional.
- The conditions of products must be at ambient temperatures.
- Have the ability to self-heal and adapt to the neighborhood.

It is necessary to combine the principles of biodesign with a systematic bioengineering approach in order to produce biomaterials that are independent of each other but must be found together. Engineers are responsible for the design and production of a biomaterial, and life scientists should be responsible for the sustainability of vital activities and adaptation to the body [35].

One of the oldest biomimicry approaches known to be designed is black boxes, hoods, and other security elements in the air using shock absorptive capability of woodpeckers. Inspired by this approach, a shock absorber material was designed by Yoon and Park [36]. This material is formed by combining one rigid surface, one viscoelastic surface, one porosity structure, and another rigid structure like a skull representation. This biomaterial designed for degeneration in regions prone to impact in the body has found many applications in the medical field (**Figure 14**).

Another important biomaterial example is "bioglass" (**Figure 15**). It is a material designed by Hench and his colleagues to replace the broken bones of soldiers who were injured during the Vietnam War [37]. CaO, P_2O_5 is added to SiO_2, and hydroxyapatite is stimulated to form different forms. By varying the ratios of the molecules, different forms can be produced. Today, there are still many varieties that are used instead of bones or that can be used as base materials for the attachment of fibrous materials.

Tissue engineering is the most used field of biomaterials. Bioengineered scaffolds are the most important biomaterials that will be used to form a tissue or an organ. Scaffolds act like the extracellular matrix in the body, aiming to attach, replicate, transform, and actively function on the cells themselves. The porosity of these biomaterials is crucial so that the cells can easily access the minimum elements to survive for life. The biomaterial must disappear when cells complete their function and become an organ in practice. For this reason, the timing of biodegradation is a very important issue that needs to be addressed [35].

Many materials can be used as biomaterial raw materials.

- Extracellular matrix (ECM).
- Biopolymers: collagen, alginate, chitosan, etc.
- Sensitive polymers; polyglyconic acid, polylactic acid, etc.
- Hydrogels, polyvinyl alcohol.
- Ceramic materials, calcium phosphate, hydroxyapetite.

Another important issue in the biomaterial production is the formation of scaffold structure. Providing high porosity and adhesion area is very important in scaffold production, solvent casting, melt molding, and 3D printing.

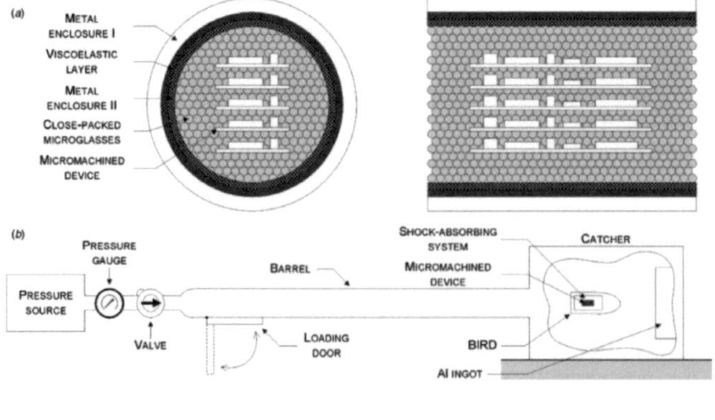

Figure 14. Bioinspired shock absorption system based on the head of the woodpecker (taken from iopscience.iop.org).

http://dx.doi.org/10.5772/intechopen.72912

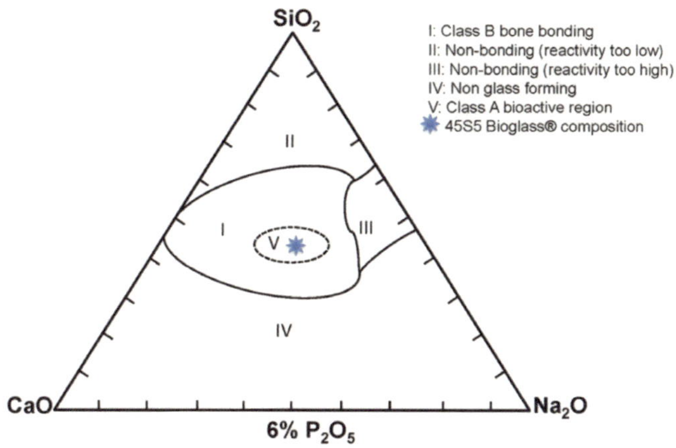

Figure 15. Bioglass composition [36].

Orthomimetics is an important biomaterial produced by Pek and the colleges [38]. It is an osteochondral scaffold. It is two sided and regenerates the bone-cartilage interphase. It is a 5 mm tape. One side includes type 1 collagen and minerals to support bone formation and the other side consists of type 2 collagen and glycosaminoglycan (GAG) to support the cartilage formation of the osteoblasts, which helps in the regeneration of bone deformations.

Biomimetic vesicles for drug delivery is very important for a controlled delivery of drug to human body. As it is known, cell boundaries are made up of a lipid barrier in which the necessary elements first dissolve in and then are released into the cell. This idea was applied to a new drug delivery system like in **Figure 16**.

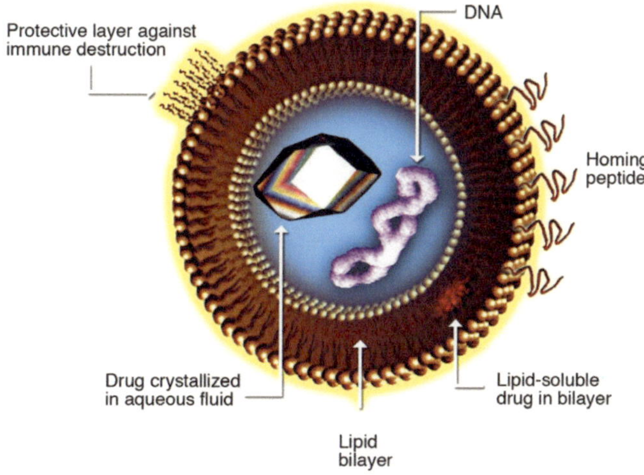

Figure 16. Liposome for drug delivery system (taken from en.wikipedia.org).

Another example of biomaterials is from cardiac studies proposed by Parker et al. In this study, artificial heart muscle prepared by 2D engineering from rat ventricular myocytes was formed. The data showed that increased systolic stress increased with increasing sarcoma compliance. Studies have suggested that the engineering process of the extracellular space is the mean of the self-organizing ability of the contractile apparatus maximizing the contractile force of cardiac myocytes. These results have significant implications for maximizing the physiological function of bioengineering tissues.

Biomimicry of the function and shape will probably result in novel treatments and to mimic such bioprocesses will be more difficult to success, but will have more effect. Another important project by Dr. Elvassore's group was developed in an in vitro cardiac tissue test, which uses human cardiomyocytes (hCMs) and microtechnologies. hCMs were grown on a polyacrylamide hydrogel with adjustable mechanical properties similar to tissues. The data showed that micromodeled hCM maintained the expression and functional properties of large cardiac markers (cTnT, cTnI, Cx43, Nkx2.5, and a-actinin). These studies are a proof that it is still a principle. However, when it is further developed, it may be an important influence on drug-based studies. As the researches in biotechnology and drug-development systems are increased, the possibility of biomimicry to take progress and take a greater role in these areas can deepen in biomedical field.

6. Future prospects

Minimum CO_2 emission technologies and sustainable solutions to the daily requirements are globally attracting the society and also the governments among developed and developing countries. Bioengineering presents a unique paradigm in various fields as a novel basis for technological thinking. It has been integrated with biomimicry through biodesign that involves nature as a massive database of mechanisms and strategies to be implemented in. Advancements in bioengineering have led to changes in biodesign approach since the last century where the terms of sustainability, environment, and ecological habitat have gained attention. The products of bacteria, fungi, and microalgal strains are generally cost effective, nontoxic, and natural, and those products can be utilized in daily-used structures/materials.

Bio-based products can be multifunctional, complex, and highly responsive solutions and thus can replace the concept of traditional strategies for a known process to improve energy performance into a new form. For example, live structural designs that use microalgae for input where buildings can adapt to changes through the environmental variations (temperature, etc.) have been realized to answer environmental concerns about greenhouse gases. This building can help future structures to be more responsive to both external and internal conditions and satisfies welfare levels for humans. However, there are still great challenges about the production of the structures planned to be built using biomimetic design approach. The transfer of knowledge and technology from bioengineers to architects is difficult. Interdisciplinary studies between those fields can employ a great role to develop bio-based products in the future.

http://dx.doi.org/10.5772/intechopen.72912

7. Conclusion

Last decades, biodesign has gained more importance because of the need in reducing environmental impacts of synthetic and chemical productions. Thus, trends in biodesign are a result of the environmental and health-related concerns. For example, using microorganisms for biocalcification instead of chemical-based concrete to make concrete self-heal would extend the service life of the concrete while lowering the costs of maintenance. As another example, the illuminating capacity of microalgae can be used in roads and pathways to increase sustainability. Fungi can also serve as a great example for their usage in decorative home products. Consequently, using technologies, designs, and models that integrate nature into bio-activity in a way that is beneficial to both ecosystem and humanity, whether by bacteria or by fungi embedded in infrastructures or algae generating our energy, may be considered as the best, smartest, and most applicable way to avoid global ecological ruin.

Author details

Irem Deniz[1]* and Tugba Keskin-Gundogdu[2]

*Address all correspondence to: iremdenz@gmail.com

1 Department of Bioengineering, Manisa Celal Bayar University, Manisa, Turkey

2 Department of Bioengineering, Ege University, Izmir, Turkey

References

[1] Beer R, Quinn R, Chiel H, Ritzmann R. Biologically inspired approaches to robotics: What can we learn from insects? CACM. 1999;**40**(3):30-38

[2] Pavlovic M. Bioengineering: A conceptual Approach. 1st ed. Heidelberg New York Dordrecht London: Springer Cham; 2015. pp. 1-13

[3] Forbes P. The Gecko's Foot: Bio-inspiration, Engineering New Materials and Devices from Nature. Harper Collins; 2005. p. 25-28

[4] Bosner R. Patented biologically-inspired technological innovations: A twenty year view. Journal of Bionic Engineering. 2006;**3**:39-41

[5] Helms M, Vattam S, Goel A. Biologically inspired design: Process and products; 2016. Design Studies. 2009;**30**:606-622

[6] Adeel Z, Bogardi J, Braeuel C, Chasek P, Niamir-Fuller N, Gabriels D, et al. Overcoming the greatest environmental challange out of our times: Re-thinking policies to cope

with desertification. In: United Nations University. International Network on Water, Environment and Health; 17-19 December 2007; Ontario, Canada. United Nations University; 2007. pp. 1-36

[7] Myers W, Antonelli P. BioDesign: Nature Science Creativity. 1st ed. Thames & Hudson, London: The Museum of Modern Art (MoMA); 2012. 288 p

[8] Turkey Biodesign Team [Internet]. 1 September 2016 [Updated: 2017]. Available from: http://www. http://www.biodesignteam.com/ [Accessed: 18.09.2017]

[9] Dosier G. Methods for making construction material using enzyme producing bacteria. Patent No: US 20110262640 A1. 2011

[10] Radeck J, Kraft K, Bartels J, Cikovic T, Dürr F, Emenegger J, et al. The bacillus BioBrick box: Generation and evaluation of essential genetic building blocks for standardized work with *Bacillus subtilis*. Journal of Biological Engineering. 2013;**7**(1):29

[11] Wiktor V, Jonkers HM. Bacteria-based concrete: From concept to market. Smart Materıals and Structures. 2016;**25**(8):1-9

[12] Nikolausz M. Microbiological options to enhance the anaerobic digestion of Lignocellulosic biomass. In: The 3rd IBBA Workshop; September 10th 2015; Malmö-Sweden. Workshop Proceesing Book. 2015. pp. 1-5

[13] Etherington R. Dezeen [Internet]. 29 October 2011 [Updated: 2016]. Available from: https://www.dezeen.com/2011/10/29/microbial-home-by-philips-design/ [Accessed: 22.06.2017]

[14] Lee S. Designboom [Internet]. 19 September 2010 [Updated: 2017]. Available from: http://www.designboom.com/design/suzanne-lee-biocouture-growing-textiles/ [Accessed: 22.06.2017]

[15] Keshk SMAS. Bacterial cellulose production and its industrial applications. Journal of Bioprocessing & Biotechniques. 2014;**4**(2):12-24

[16] Kim TH, Jung SH, Choc KH. Investigations into the design principles in the chemotactic behavior of *Escherichia coli*. Bio Systems. 2012;**91**:171-182

[17] Mata TM, Martins AA. Microalgae for biodiesel production and other applications: A review. Renewable and Sustainable Energy Reviews. 2010;**14**:217-232

[18] Miklosi A. Chlorella Oxygen Pavilion Concept and the Symbiosis in Design. School of Design and Crafts, University of Gothenburg Degree Project. 2012: 48 pp

[19] Roedel C, Petersen JP. Smart Material House BIQ. International Building Exhibition Hamburg; July 2013; Hamburg. IBA Hamburg GmbH; 2013. pp. 1-22

[20] Stevermer T. Tylerstevermer [Internet]. 9 October 2014 [Updated: 2016]. Available from: https://tylerstevermer.wordpress.com/2014/09/10/algaevator/ [Accessed: 22.06.2017]

[21] Cilento K. Archdaily [Internet]. 5 September 2012 [Updated: 2017]. Available from: http://www.archdaily.com/270592/al-bahar-towers-responsive-facade-aedas [Accessed: 22.06.2017]

[22] Kim KH. A Feasibility Study of an Algae Façade System. International Conference on Sustainable Building Asia; 8-10 July 2013; Seoul- South Korea. Korea Green Building Council; 2013. pp. 333-341

[23] Grozdanic L. Evolo [Internet]. 24 February 2012 [Updated: 2017]. Available from: http://www.evolo.us/architecture/algae-urban-farm-ecologicstudio/ [Accessed: 22.06.2017]

[24] Kim KH. Beyond Green: Growing Algae Façade. Beyond Green: Bio-reactor Integrated Building Envelope (BIBE) in Urban Environment; August 2013; North Carolina. United States Environmental Protection Agency; 2013. pp. 1-16

[25] Sivasubramanian V. Environmental Sustainability Using Green Technologies. 1st ed. India: CRC Press; 2016. 430 p

[26] Watkinson S, Boddy L, Money N. The Fungi. 3rd ed. Oxford-UK: Elsevier Academic Press; 2015. 466 p

[27] Hy-Fi The Living. Biodesignchallenge [Internet]. 2017. [Updated: 2017]. Available from: http://biodesignchallenge.org/themes/architecture/ [Accessed: 22.06.2017]

[28] Mok K. Treehugger [Internet]. 23 October 2013. [Updated: 2017]. Available from: https://www.treehugger.com/eco-friendly-furniture/mycelium-chair-3d-printed-living-fungus-eric-klarenbeek.html [Accessed: 22.06.2017]

[29] Erden S. Techin2b [Internet]. 2015. [Updated: 2015]. Available from: http://www.techin2b.com/techdisplay.php?profile_id=TaE9Z2BCHx1F&&log= [Accessed: 22.06.2017]

[30] Wang L. Inhabitat [Internet]. 1 January 2016. [Updated: 2016]. Available from: http://inhabitat.com/pollution-free-furniture-of-the-future-will-be-grown-from-mushrooms/ [Accessed: 22.06.2017]

[31] Adamatzky A. Thirty seven things to do with live slime mould. In: Advances in Unconventional Computing Volume 23 of the Series Emergence, Complexity and Computation. 1st ed. UK: Springer; 2016. pp. 709-738

[32] Tero A, Takagi S, Saigusa T, Ito K, Bebber DP, Fricker MD, et al. Rules for biologically inspired adaptive network design. Science. 2010;**327**(5964):439-442

[33] Nimgaonkar A, Yock P, Brinton T, Krummel T, Pasricha P. Gastroenterology and biodesign: Contributing to the future of our specialty. Gastroenterology. 2013;**144**:258-262

[34] Bryskin A, Brown AC, Baksh M,, Finn M.G. Barker T.Learning from nature—Novel synthetic biology approaches for biomaterial design. Acta Biomaterialia. 2014;**10**:1761-1769

[35] Chen PY, McKittrick J, Meyers MA. Biological materials: Functional adaptations and bioinspired designs. Progress in Materials Science. 2012;**57**:1492-1704

[36] Yoon S-H, Park S. A mechanical analysis of woodpecker drumming and its application to shock-absorbing systems. Bioinspiration and Biomimicry. 2011;**6**:1-12

[37] Hench LL. The story of Bioglass. Journal of Materials Science. Materials in Medicine. 2006;**17**:967-978

[38] Pek YS, Spector M, Yanna IV, Gibson LJ. Degradation of a collagen-chondroitin-6 sulfate matrix by collagenase and chondroitinase. Biomaterials. 2004;**25**:472-482

Chapter 5

Biomimetic Facade Applications for a More Sustainable Future

Ayça Tokuç, Fatma Feyzal Özkaban and
Özge Andiç Çakır

Additional information is available at the end of the chapter

http://dx.doi.org/10.5772/intechopen.73021

Abstract

Mankind has often taken inspiration from the nature to solve problems since nature has sophisticated processes, refined for thousands of years. While manmade systems are unsustainable, natural processes embody sustainability principles; therefore, there are many things to learn from nature in order to solve design problems and create a more sustainable future. This is the promise of a biomimetic design approach. Another design approach is biodesign, and it also involves utilizing natural elements inside the design. The building façade is a problematic research area since it is at the intersection between living spaces and natural environment; thus it faces many problems especially regarding energy-air-water transition between indoors and outdoors. Application of key sustainability concepts in architecture such as energy requirements, form and structure, and sustainability considerations can be enhanced by learning from natural processes. This chapter looks at cutting-edge design principles, materials, and designs in building façades through the lens of biomimetics and biodesign. First, the design principles and then the materials and some cases are explained. The concepts of biomimicry and biodesign are in harmony with the concept of sustainability; however, to reach sustainable façade solutions, the sustainability principles should be at the core of the design problem definition.

Keywords: adaptive façade, biomimetics, biodesign, construction materials, sustainable architecture

1. Introduction

The relationship between nature, technology, and architecture is an ancient debate with many historical twists and turns; however, these past decades have brought unprecedentedly quick paradigm shifts. Biomimicry is a relatively new term, yet its connotations have been part of architecture for millennia, especially in form generation and imitating structural systems. While our interpretation for the earliest works is mostly conjecture, the written works relate the architectural styles of art nouveau, streamline design, anthropomorphism, zoomorphism, biomorphism, organic design, and biologically inspired design as precursors to biomimetics, biomimesis, or bionic [1]. While some designers and researchers interpret biomimicry as an all-encompassing approach to learn from nature (such as the biomimicry institute), others argue it should only be used to identify mimicking biological processes, and other phenomena should be called by different names. These include biophilia (love of nature) for taking inspiration from natural forms [2], biomimesis for imitation of natural models and systems, and geomimicry for utilizing geological processes instead of biological ones.

One of the recent innovation areas is material sciences, such as new ways of making old materials and innovation at nanoscales. Biomimicry processes tend to be either problem based, from design problem to biology, or solution based, from biology to design [3]. A newer term is biodesign; it encompasses mimicking biological processes; moreover it also includes integrating biological organisms as a part of the design or construction processes. Recent innovation areas include redesigning construction methods and material sciences by making use of biological materials. While there are few built examples, biodesign continues to evolve and utilizes both a problem-based approach and a solution-based approach simultaneously.

In this period of paradigm shifts, Benyus' definition of the role of architecture as creating environments inductive to human life [4] is also evolving. The debates on environmental impact and sustainability influence architecture through the world with new codes and measures; these are most visible on the topics of energy efficiency and environmental impact of buildings during and after construction. However, human-made environments and architectural systems are not sustainable since they make use of land, require resource inputs, and generate waste products. Therefore, architectural practices continue to search for more sustainable design concepts; some of the common concepts include passive, active, energy-efficient, zero energy, green, and intelligent. Yet all sustainable design concepts place an essential role to the building façade design since its place at the intersection between living spaces and natural environment makes it the skin of the building, where energy-air-water transition between indoors and outdoors occurs.

The main performance criteria of a sustainable façade include "energy requirements," "form and structure," and "sustainability considerations." Although all nature-inspired designs are not sustainable, this chapter argues that architects and engineers can employ biodesign principles for higher performing façades. In this context, this chapter aims to investigate the possibilities of biomimetics and biodesign methods in sustainability of constructional practices of the future, façades in particular. The scope is looking at design parameters, materials, and state of the art in building façades from a biomimetic and biodesign point of view. Although the number of materials and examples given in this study are limited in number, they put forward the given principles. This paper first discusses the design principles of sustainable façades, then explains related construction materials, and afterward investigates examples.

http://dx.doi.org/10.5772/intechopen.73021

2. Design parameters for sustainable biomimetic façades

Façade is the exterior element of the building that separates the indoors and outdoors, yet another significant role of a façade is giving image to the building. Façades perform under the influence of climate conditions and affect the indoor living conditions; therefore the first criteria of a sustainable façade are usually defined as material and energy efficiency (**Figure 1**). Architects and engineers employ thermal, optical, air flow, and electrical mechanisms for higher performance in façades. Aksamija defines high-performance sustainable façades as exterior enclosures that use the least possible amount of energy to maintain a comfortable interior environment, which promotes the health and productivity of the building's occupants [5].

In this context, biomimetics and biodesign have helped to create façades for a long time; however, all designs that take nature into consideration are not sustainable. To create a sustainable façade, the design constraints should take into account the parameters for sustainable living models, for instance, how do organisms heat, cool, give shade, and control light?

A sustainable design problem would treat an organic skin as animated by natural phenomena, i.e., wind, light, rain, drought, snow, etc. In addition, it can also perform other functions

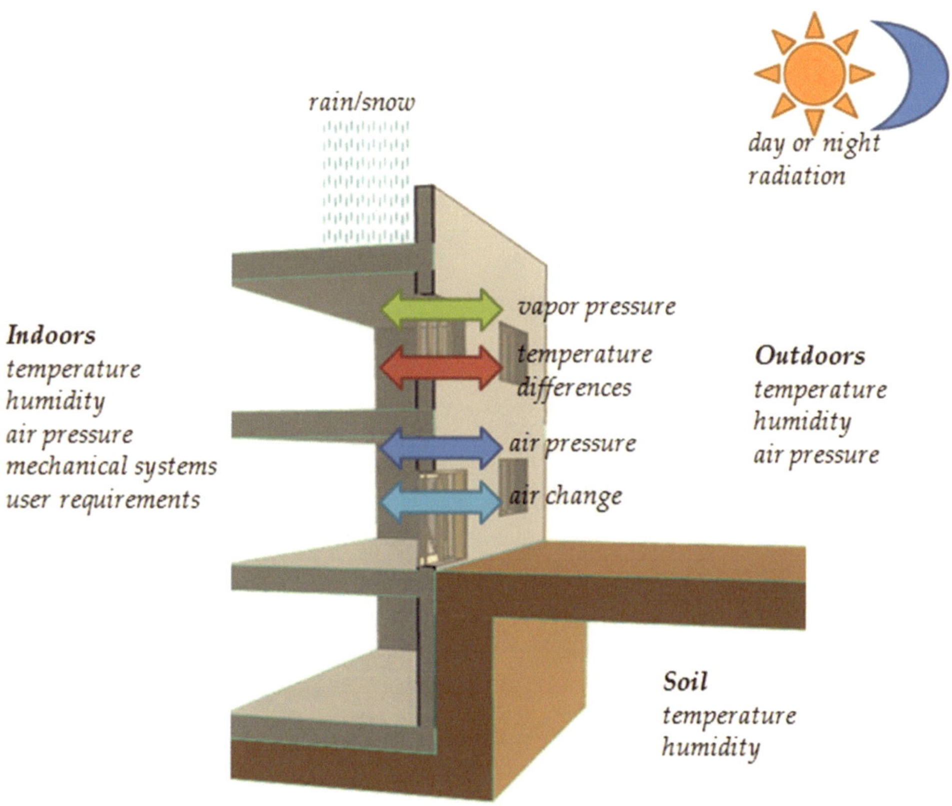

Figure 1. Design principles of a traditional facade, by TBT, 2017.

essential to life such as breathing, carbon capture, and water balance; for such functionality they usually have multiple layers. Loonen describes the underlying principles of bio-inspired façade design as adaptability, multi-ability, and evolvability [6]. **Figure 2** schematically represents the main design principles for a sustainable façade. Thus energy requirements, functional considerations, and structural efficiency should be integrated in a more sustainable façade.

2.1. Energy requirements

The most common design metric for sustainability of buildings is energy requirement to regulate the indoor environmental conditions. Most of the energy consumed in a building is necessary for heating/cooling requirements and is directly related to the façade design, since most of heat and light transfer between indoors and outdoors takes place through the façade. The regulation of time-dependent weather data such as solar irradiation, ambient temperature, sky temperature, wind speed, and relative humidity is necessary. From a sustainability point of view, these technologies can be classified under thermal comfort, visual comfort, and renewable energy production.

The parameters related to heat and energy transfer are solar radiation, wind, and climate. The utilization of a façade for thermal comfort changes according to the properties and thickness of the material layers in addition to the heat balance on the element's surface due to both the properties of the materials (i.e., thermal absorption, emissivity, density, specific heat, and

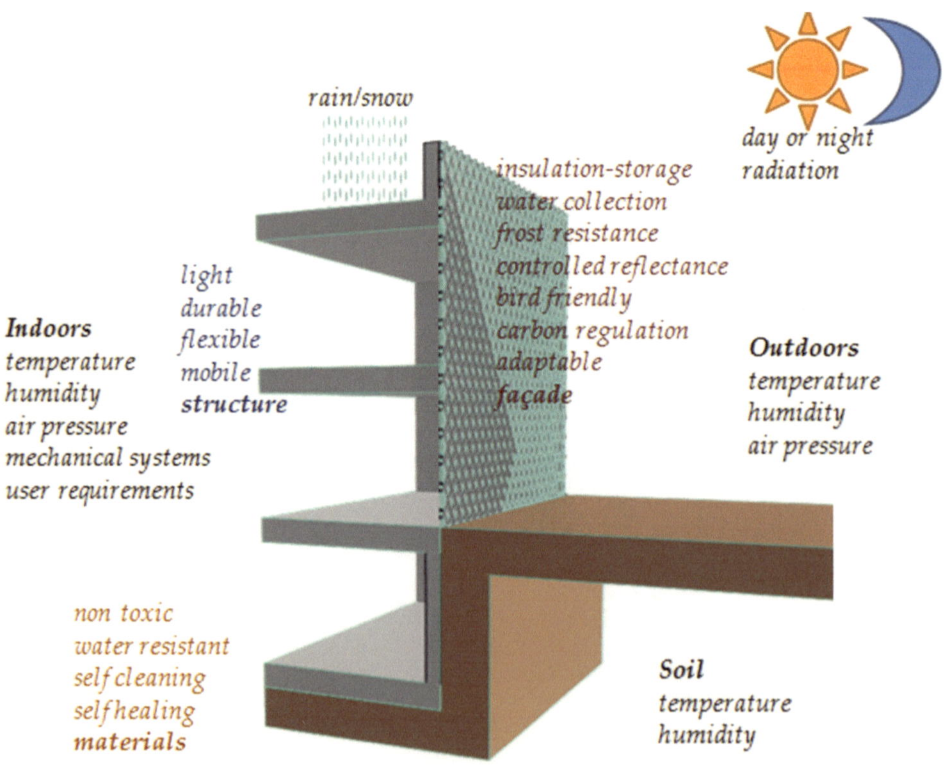

Figure 2. Design principles of a sustainable facade, by TBT, 2017.

thermal conductivity). These are usually regulated with architectural technologies including solar orientation, insulation, and shading. In addition, there are a number of less common dynamic technologies such as thermal mass, dynamic insulation, radiative cooling, phase change, energy storage, natural ventilation, and energy generation.

TRIZ is a Russian acronym for theory of inventive problem solving, while BioTRIZ is a methodology that can interpret and transfer data from biology into technological procedures. Craig et al. used BioTRIZ to design a roof for a hot climate, Arabia [7]. The problem involves conventional roof design with high thermal insulation that would prohibit solar radiation and convection effects from warming the thermal mass of the roof yet at the same time restrict its radiative cooling. While many solutions were offered by the methodology, the researchers chose to replace the existing insulation with an open cell honeycomb that would stop convective warming yet at the same time allow long wave radiation to pass vertically. They estimate a reduction of surface temperature by an average of 4.5°C.

Visual comfort depends on the amount of necessary light and lack of glare. Levels of light transmission, transparency, translucency, color, and reflection effect interior-exterior light transmission and indoor lighting conditions. While glass systems that respond to light, electricity, and heat exist, the homeostatic façade system used by architecture firm Decker Yeadon mimics the muscle system and uses electrochemistry to lengthen and contract the dielectric elastomer to create a self-shading glass [8].

The façades can become generators of renewable energy. The primary energy source on earth is photosynthesis, which became the precursor for fossil fuels. Today photovoltaic technology biomimics plants to create artificial photosynthesis [9]. Some façades can be used to cultivate or act in mutual coordination with species such as algae that can grow and be harvested for oil, so they are suitable as a biodiesel, bioethanol, bio-hydrogen, or biomass production source (see Section 4.4). Yet these need not be living organisms and can be systems mimicking living organisms such as building integrated nano-wind turbines [10].

2.2. Form and structural efficiency

The most common type of biomimicry in architecture is copying surface morphology from nature. There are lots of buildings that take their shapes from nature, from bones to leaves and flowers to shells. Sometimes the analogy is only morphologic, as in the iconic Sydney Opera House's analogy with an orange shell, yet sometimes the appearance also serves a purpose. For instance, the roof of Esplanade Theaters in Singapore by DP Architects uses durian fruit as a model and their spikes as inspiration for sun shading and likewise has a secondary sun shading lattice; thus, it captures the sun, reduces its energy use, and reduces artificial lighting [11].

While most discourses on architecture emphasize that biological data will cause changes in architectural paradigms, most of the studies are focused on form generation [12]. Today, complex geometries can be defined by a set of rules for growth in parametric terms using computational methods. Gruber et al. propose a multistage design process that aim to address strategic decisions at the start of a project while facilitating exploration of architectural design. The stages of this process are identifying the features of the design; extracting feature genes; generating the new evolved and developed typology, i.e., phenotype; and altering genes to modify the phenotype [13].

While utilization of evolutionary algorithms in parametric design is a widely discussed research topic, another aspect of digital technology in architecture is making entirely digital fabrication possible via CNC or 3D printing for these complex geometries. This would allow for material efficiency and ease of fabrication yet continue to be biomimetic. Yet minimal carbon footprint is only possible with an efficiently designed structure that is stable and durable and makes use of its environment to have minimal impact. Inspiration from biological processes and implementation of nature's principles allows for the design of façades in alignment with the flow of forces according to nature of the structure itself.

Through history, most of the structural systems were thus influenced from nature. From the cave houses to tensile structures, the prototypes of structural systems surround us through nature. Some of the earlier structural system classifications take these into account. The biomimetic approach looks at and sees insect mound in the masonry structures such as pyramids, shell structures in eggshells, tensile structures in spider webs, cell structures in honeycombs, and pneumatics in soap bubbles [14]. The first studies that emphasize that biomimicry is not only formal analogical but have to be an inspirational process from nature began in the early twentieth century and spread.

Some examples include Dischinger's reinforced concrete dome for shells (**Figure 3a**), Buckminster Fuller's revolutionary geodesic dome construction for space frame construction (**Figure 3b**), and Frei Otto's work on lightweight construction for tensile structures. In recent studies, the façade of One Ocean Pavilion by SOMA Architecture and Knippers Helbig Engineering for Yeosu Expo 2012 looks like fish gills from the outside, yet the hingeless structure of the lamellas that also regulate the light and air inside was inspired by the opening mechanism of the bird of paradise flower [15] (see Section 4.2). Thus bio-kinematics can be transferred to technical constructions to create ever-changing surfaces.

2.3. Sustainability considerations

Scientific research suggests that anthropogenic carbon emissions lie at the heart of global warming, yet nature uses carbon as a building element of living organisms. An essential issue of architectural processes is the utilization of optimum amount of resources and thus has lower ecological footprints. Moreover, nature also has no waste since output of one process serves as input for another. In addition, the chemical reactions in natural processes require neither high temperatures nor toxicity [4]. Another point is that while manmade environments mainly

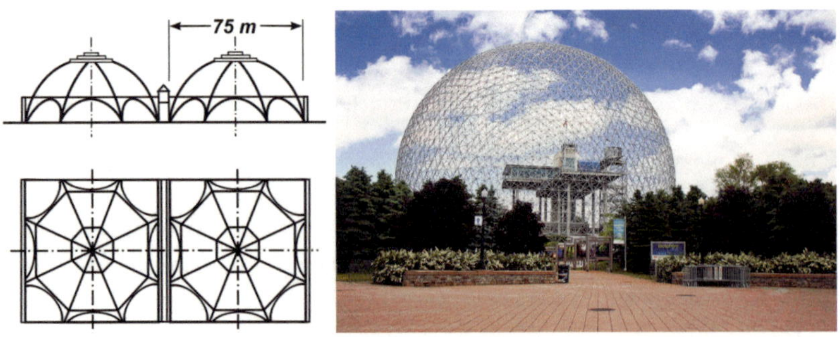

Figure 3. Biomimetic structural examples; (left) reinforced concrete dome [16] and (right) geodesic dome [17].

rely on outside energy sources, the main energy source of nature is the sun and gravity. In this way, nature has various clues to offer humans for a more sustainable life. The façades also serve many considerations including air quality, water efficiency, carbon capture, use of nontoxic materials, low embodied energy, low material consumption, biological behavior, responsive, adaptable, breathing, and sensing.

Photosynthesizing or fog eating façades allow for carbon sequestration from the environment (see Section 4.3). While they create more air to breathe, they may also allow breathing by the planted greenery. In addition, greenery regulates flows of heat, air, water, and electricity to maximize energy efficiency. Besides thermal comfort, indoor air quality is directly associated with health and productivity issues in buildings [18]. The façade in Council House 2 by Mick Pierce in Melbourne makes use of a number of biomimetic principles to manage heating, lighting, air quality, and water inside the building. Every aspect of the building has been rethought so as to function as a tree with eco-tech architectural technologies. The façade is multilayered like the human skin; the outer skin (dermis) consists of stairs, ducts, balconies, sunscreens, and foliage for solar and glare control and creates a semi-enclosed microclimate [19].

Water is the source of life on Planet Earth, and it is the living medium for many organisms, yet in a building, the water considerations are twofold. First is the protection from water, and second is the efficient use of fresh water for resource conservation. Badarnah and Kadri propose the BioGen methodology for biomimetic design concept generation. It focuses on investigation of integrating a number of strategies to achieve improved solutions [20]. They use this methodology on the design problem for a water-harvesting façade in arid regions. First they map their exploration in a graph for four hierarchical levels: function, process, factors, and pinnacles that inhabit the region. Then they define pathways on the map, select from pinnacles, analyze, and classify selected pinnacles in order to reduce complexity. The dominant features in each category are identified and superposed with the design paths. The resulting preliminary design is based on the Thorny Devil (**Figure 4**), which is one of the many pinnacles in the system. The design includes a bumpy surface that attracts the water molecules, and grooves generated between the mounds that encourage capillary action into storage chambers. The water in the chambers is then transported through the wall and evaporated inside. They estimate that the wall would humidify the interior for one third of the year.

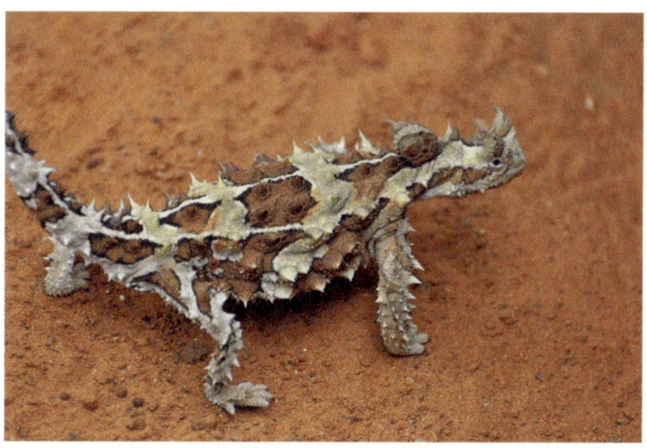

Figure 4. The thorny devil [21].

3. Biomimetic building materials and techniques for façade applications

Today, the building façade is no longer a cover to only protect the structure from the outside environment. The design of a façade aims to impart functional characteristics as well as an esthetic look; in addition, it considers extending the life of the building with more durable materials. Thus, a façade may be designed as an adaptive layer which has a great impact on the energy efficiency and thermal comfort of the whole building. With an interdisciplinary approach, stronger, functional, durable, and ecologically efficient building façades may be designed.

Bio-inspired manufacturing, either in micro-, nano-, or macro-level, manufacturing of materials or systems derived from biological self-organization methods, i.e., self-healing, self-cleaning, and self-assembly, are efficiently used for these purposes. Biological organisms themselves may be enforced to live and produce in a manmade environment, and their efficient characteristics are engineered; examples of those include fungi-producing thermal insulation materials for energy-efficient façades or algal photobioreceptors for energy generation.

The interdisciplinary approach for using microorganisms and/or their products may be termed as "microbial biotechnology" or as a more generic name "construction bioengineering." Bio-inspired climate adaptive building skins that behave like a living organism may create an ecosystem that can provide a mutual relationship with the outdoor environment [22]. As an example of green walls, the biological materials such as greenery can be used as a material to cover a façade and to control temperature variations [23].

Either on organism, behavior, or ecosystem level, when inspiration comes from nature, it may reflect in various ways in building façades: designing a functional or esthetic form; producing a functional material for building the façade; adding a novel function, e.g., self-cleaning or energy saving; and constructing the façade with a new technique. Sometimes a biomimetic process may be used to produce the façade-making materials (**Figure 5**).

One may classify the biomimetic solutions for construction purposes by observing the examples available and researching the novel techniques that are still in the initial technology readiness levels. However, a deeper question arises, "why do we need biomimetic solutions for building façade applications?" Structural and functional necessities as well as rising importance on sustainability and energy efficiency divert scientists and engineers working on construction materials field to biomimetic solutions (**Figure 6**).

Regarding the necessities described above, there are many novel solutions based on interdisciplinary to transdisciplinary works. Some examples of façade-making construction materials and techniques are described below.

The high contact angle between the surface and the liquid-air interface of some plants, such as lotus, results in hydrophobic surfaces; those surfaces have self-cleaning ability as the water drops may slip easily carrying the contaminants away from the surface [24]. Gecko feet [25], pond skater [26], and shark skin [27] are other examples that human inspire for producing functional surfaces. These natural mechanisms were applied by construction industry to many products such as self-cleaning paints or clay roof tiles; in addition textile and automotive

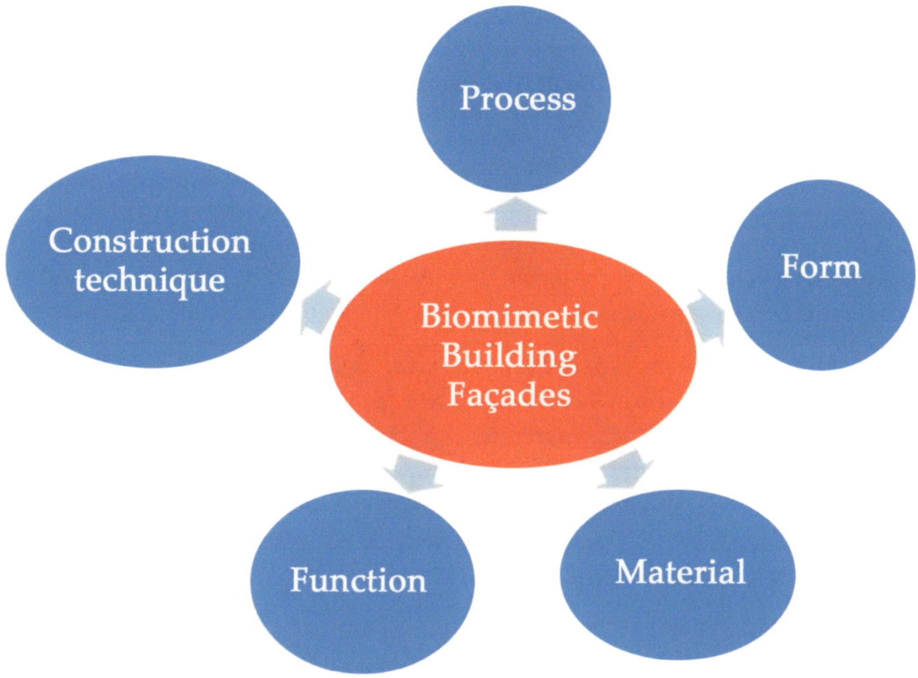

Figure 5. Biomimetic technologies for building facade design, by TBT, 2017.

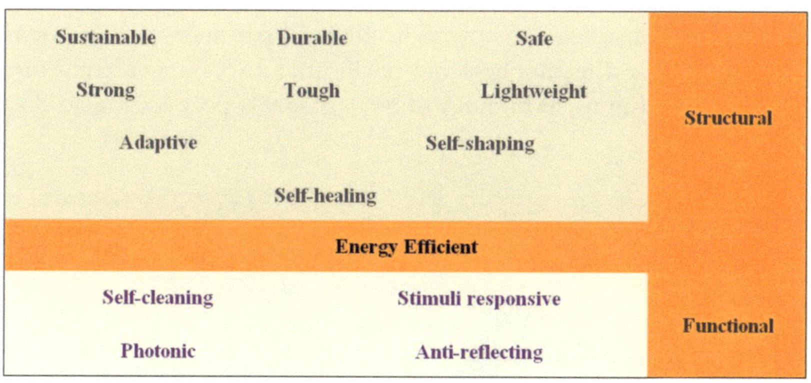

Figure 6. Biomimetic solutions for construction materials used in facades, by TBT, 2017.

industry has produced similar solutions. Inspired from photosynthesis process, photocatalytic effects work in the combination of air humidity, UV radiation, oxygen, and nanoscale catalyst TiO_2 being a basis for industrial self-cleaning paints and other industrial applications [28]. Having some commercial examples available, photocatalytic TiO_2 nanoparticles are able to clean air of automobile-produced nitrogen oxides (NO_X), providing them with extra functionality [29] (see Section 4.3).

Anti-reflectivity is an important functionality for surfaces that may be useful for energy-efficient façade applications. The eyes of the elephant hawk moth are coated with a regular pattern of conical nanoprotuberances, which significantly minimize light reflection. This ability improves night vision and is critical for moths to escape predators. Nanostructured moth-eye arrays are optically excellent for reducing reflections and used for applications such as glazing the skyscrapers and silicon solar cells [30, 31].

Inspired from the organisms living in arid climates, phase-changing materials store energy during melting and freezing. By using the thermal insulation materials for façade applications, interior spaces stay cool (or warm) for a longer period of time improving energy efficiency [32, 33].

Cultivation of living matter on façades is not a novel idea, and the green walls are a part of everyday architecture; however, when it comes to adding microalgae photobioreactor to the façade of a building, the benefits differentiate, and the process becomes more complex. Algae capture the energy by photosynthesis inside the open or closed systems that contain water, nutrients, and CO_2. Those systems can be integrated on the façade of a building through convenient designs that provide necessary sunlight for algae growth. Integrated photo-bioreactor solutions enable energy efficiency for both buildings and cities [34, 35].

The biological formation of minerals, i.e., biomineralization process, in particular the biocalcification, is used to form bio-binders, hardening sand to gain new forms, healing cracks in reinforced concrete buildings, soil stabilization and environmental processes, etc. It is possible to produce microbial (or bacterial) binders by microbial-induced calcium carbonate precipitation, thus producing novel materials for construction and enhancing their durability [36]. A commercial example of this is a technique patented by Dosier and labeled as BioMason™. The Biodesign Team Turkey (TBT) aimed to develop architectural design product that is in harmony with the nature and suitable to human health with partnership of bioengineering and architecture disciplines via directing bacterial calcification to form an architectural structure with the support of 3D printing technology of biodegradable poly-lactic acid (PLA). For this

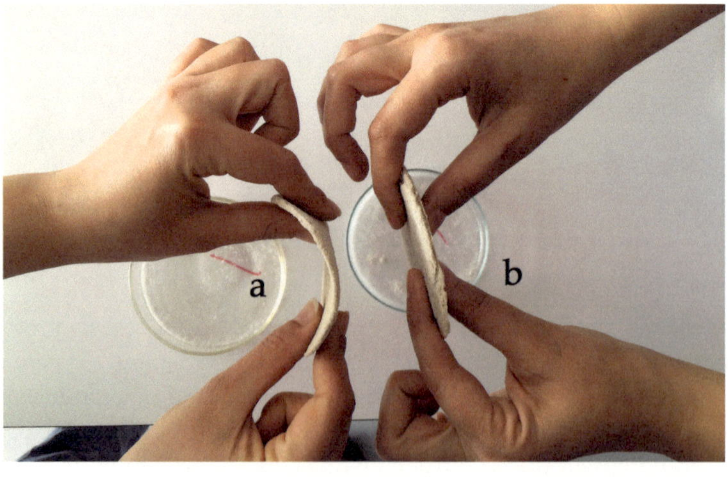

Figure 7. Solidification trials on petri dishes ((a) without inoculum; (b) with inoculum), by TBT, 2017.

http://dx.doi.org/10.5772/intechopen.73021

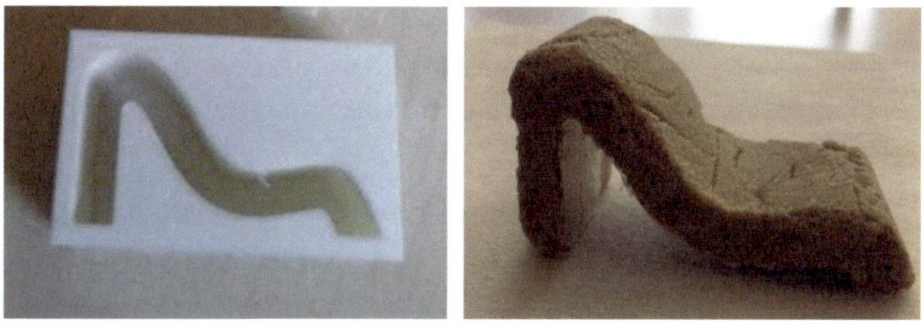

Figure 8. Prototype seating element: (left) 3D-printed design and (right) solidified urban unit, by TBT, 2017.

purpose, *Sporosarcina pasteurii* (*Bacillus pasteurii*) was chosen to use the urea mechanism to precipitate $CaCO_3$, thus hardening sand by utilizing urea (**Figure 7**).

After the successful solidification process in petri dishes, a unique life element was designed, and the mold was taken out from the 3D printer (**Figure 8** (left)). The mold was covered with sand, and then inoculum was added and evenly distributed throughout. The DSM 33 growth medium containing 100 mM $CaCl_2$ was evenly distributed on the sand too and incubated for 1 week in a 30°C incubator. The lab-type prototype (**Figure 8** (right)) shows that real scale designs can be produced harmless, and environment-friendly life elements at large scales can be produced.

In addition, embedding the microbial agents in cement matrix by several methods, which may improve the microstructure of the material, furthermore, they may impart self-healing ability to such systems by bacterial biocalcium carbonate formation as a natural mechanism. Self-healing

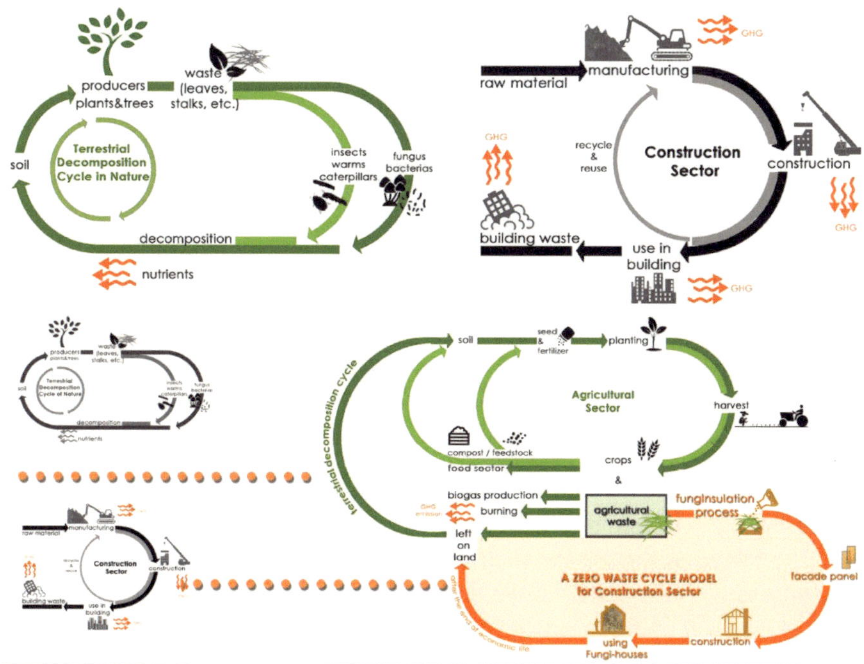

Figure 9. Funginsulation architecture concept; (upper left) decomposition cycle in nature, (upper right) Lifecycle, and (down) funginsulation cycle, by TBT and Diploid, 2017.

is a mechanism of living organisms. Various methodologies such as usage of hollow fibers and pipettes resembling the veins in living organisms, incorporation of encapsulated agents, and implementation of expansive agents, mineral admixtures, and bacteria have been employed to tackle the vulnerability of cementitious materials to cracks [37] by a self-healing mechanism.

The ability to grow fungi by producing mycelium is the functionalized part of FungInsulation™ concept. A mycelium is a vegetative part of fungus, and it consists of branching mass named hyphae. Fungal mycelium can spread over soil and many other substrates by using the nutrients inside [38].

Rural Funginsulation Architecture concept by TBT and Diploid is a value-added solution to recycle agricultural waste to design and energy efficiently retrofit rural houses. A bio-inspired process is used to produce construction materials with superior thermal insulation property, and the solutions are tailor-designed for several rural areas having different agricultural waste types (**Figure 9**).

The abovementioned materials and techniques developed by biomimetic concept are examples of sustainable and functional solutions. Many others are under development, and they will provide more energy-efficient, durable, and functional solutions in the future. Thus, building skins with adaptive capabilities approaching to that of natural skins are on the way.

4. Contemporary biomimetic façade applications

According to Benyus' classification [4], biomimicry can mimic natural forms and natural processes. Designers can imitate the features of creatures or their behaviors. However, there are also cases of another level of biological inspiration, a bio-collaborative design that makes use of living organisms in the façade design. Below are some examples that make use of the aforementioned design principles and materials to generate various designs.

4.1. Experimental smartness

Media-TIC (1997–2007) is an office building designed by Enric Ruiz-Geli (from Cloud 9 architects) for Consorci de la Zona Franca and located in 22@ of Barcelona Poble Nou district, at the intersection of Carrer Roc Boronat and Carrer Sancho de Ávila. The 22@ is a science and technological district, which was converted from the old industrial area of the city, and is continuing to transform with many experimental high-tech buildings since 2000. In this environment, Media-tic building is named as "a kind of house of the Digital Community" and could be seen as a technological showcase that serves the purpose of being "green smart city" of Barcelona.

The building was designed exclusively using CAD/CAM technology. The design approach of Cloud 9 sanctifies the technology, and they regard Media-TIC as true representative of the digital age: "The theme of the Media-TIC building is how architecture creates a new balance with the digital use of energy… now we are undergoing the DIGITAL revolution. Between 1900-1950 the cathedrals of architecture were built: these were the factories. Factories whose technological and structural advances created work spaces. In the information era, architecture has to be a technological platform, in which bits, connectivity, new materials and nanotechnology are important." They describe this design as "performative architecture" where the structure itself performs other functions [39].

This building has a hybrid program and proposes an information and communications technology center. The ground floor contains an open space and a communications hub open to the public, reception offices, and a restaurant. The building program also has an auditorium for 300 people on the first floor and offices, with open and flexible floor plans.

It can be said that Media-TIC building imitates nature's adaptability through its smart façades. The most apparent characteristic of this 38-m-high building is its adaptive architectural envelope inspired by breathing. This envelope includes "performative" elements on two of the four façades, which are made of the ethylene tetrafluoroethylene (ETFE) cladding within a net-like steel structure. ETFE was selected for its lightness, elasticity, geometrical flexibility, and thinness. The ETFE cladding surface also gives reference to the geometrical forms of atoms or elements with its concave and convex triangles. The Southeast and the Southwest façades are adaptive ETFE surfaces; their skin changes depending on the external conditions (**Figure 10**).

ETFE façades both filter out ultraviolet light and react to the changing weather conditions. On the southeast elevation, which would absorb 6 h of sunlight a day, 104 inflatable cushions are controlled by an independent computerized sensor. Each cushion contains three air chambers—a transparent outer layer, a middle layer, and third layer with a reverse pattern design. The air chambers between different layers not only slightly improve thermal insulation but also enable the control of solar radiation through a pneumatic system and a pressure sensor located in each cushion. The air inside each cushion is managed individually through a lighting sensor. It can also be manipulated and scheduled with an IP address [41]. When the sun's rays reach certain strength, air is pumped into the inner chamber and creates an opaque façade that protects the structure from the sun. When the middle and inner layers come together, they create, and the inflatable section only has one air chamber. This movement gives reference to orientation. The southwest façade consists of two ETFE sheets filled with nitrogen and oil coalescence to provide the necessary shading. This shading varies depending on the density of the air in order to obtain the desired solar transmittance [41].

The remaining façades would receive only 3 h of sunlight a day and use internal screen-type blinds for solar protection. In all, the project uses 2500 m^2 of ETFE cladding, achieving energy savings of 20%. It does not need cleaning because of the nonstick quality of the surface. It is proven to be compliant with international fire safety standards, and it does not contribute to the spread of flames or the production of smoke [41]. The building has additional sustainability goals such as a photovoltaic roof, which produces half of the

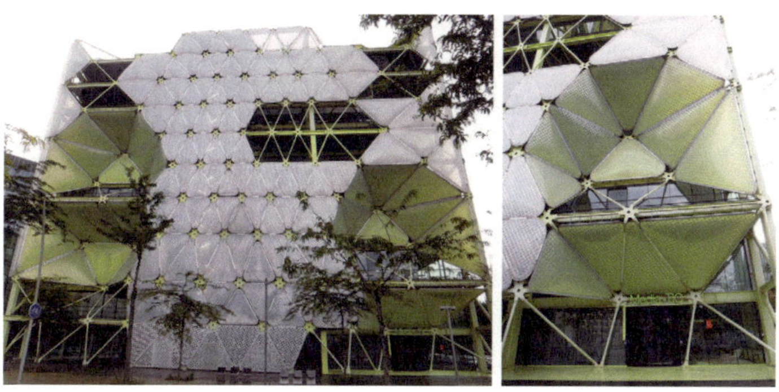

Figure 10. Media-TIC building: (left) exterior view and (right) inflatable cushions [40].

building's energy, and rainwater storage for use in the WCs. Accordingly, the building cut its emissions by 60% and gained a LEED gold certificate.

The building won World Building of the Year 2011 award in accordance with its values of 1–20% CO_2 reduction due to the use of district cooling, 2–10% CO_2 reduction due to its photovoltaic roof, 3–55% CO_2 reduction due to the dynamic ETFE sun filters, and 4–10% CO_2 reduction due to energy efficiency related to smart sensors. The building has another biomimetic approach indoors. Inspired by jellyfish, the interior paint absorbs energy from the sun all day and releases a green glow throughout the night. "It is a building that lights itself, but it does not light up the whole neighborhood" says Ruiz-Geli [39].

4.2. Kinetic façade

One Ocean Pavilion (2010–2012) was designed by SOMA Architects for an open international architecture competition regarding Expo Yeosu 2012 in South Korea. The concept of the building is based on the Expo's theme, "The Living Ocean and Coast," and emphasizes the experience of the ocean: "as an endless surface and in an immersed perspective as depth." The building has two sides; one of them meets the coastline and creates a soft meandering edge. The opposite side embraces the ocean with vertical cones and its roof landscapes (**Figure 11**).

The building owes its main concept and popularity to its kinetic façade with fish-like characteristics: "(our architectural intention is) to produce a choreography and imagery out of the building's own layers, without displaying any further media content …By involving real movement the kinetic façade aims to unify those usually isolated layers of architecture and media and define it as an interrelated and inseparable three-dimensional experience" [43].

A biomimetic approach was implemented for the kinetic façade on the main entrance façade of the building; it was developed with Knippers Helbig Engineers. The working mechanism of the façade was inspired by opening movement of the petal found in the "perch" of the bird of paradise flower (*Strelitzia reginae*) (**Figure 12**) [45], which is based on a torsional bending mechanism. Biomechanical investigations have established that the perch of the bird of paradise flower, which protects the stamen and ovary, can be released more than 3000 times with

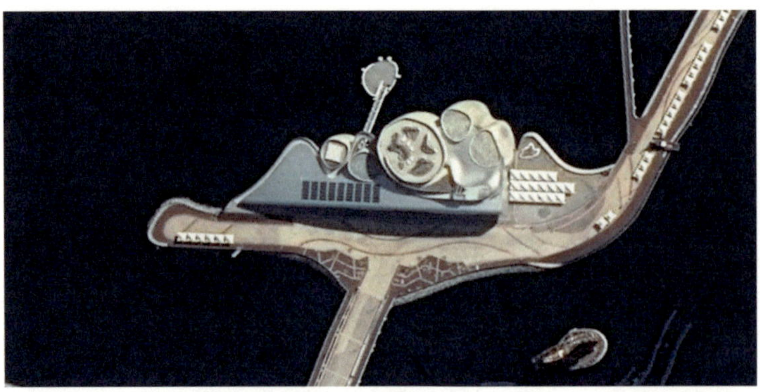

Figure 11. One Ocean Pavilion bird's eye view [42].

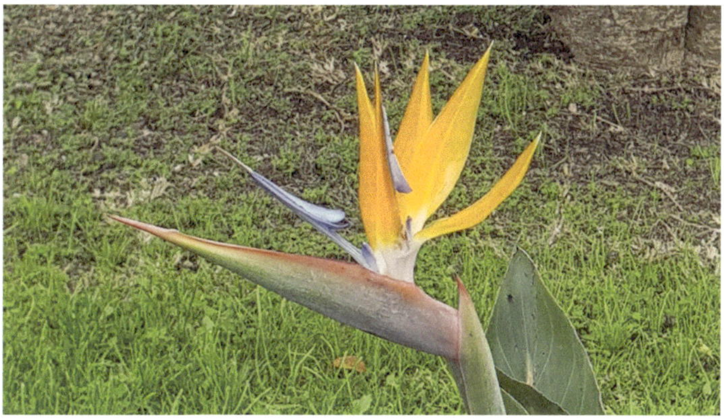

Figure 12. Bird of paradise flower, by TBT, 2018.

no evidence of fatigue [15]. When the flower is pollinated by birds, the perch is bent downward and opened by torsional buckling [44].

The kinetic façade of One Ocean building has 108 fiberglass lamellas made of glass fiber-reinforced polymers (GFRP) that open and close via a servomotor and covers a length around 140 m with a height changing from 3 m to 13 m. Slightly curved lamellas are only 9 mm thick yet can reach 14 m of length. A local compression force at the top and the bottom leads to a controlled buckling and reversible elastic deformation inside the fins [15]. Each individual modular lamella is moved by actuators located on the upper and lower edges of the façade and is operated by solar panels located on the roof. The GFRP wings undergo lateral-torsional buckling, in order to deploy into a doubly curved shape. The high strength of the glass fibers is combined with a highly flexible epoxy resin in order to achieve a low bending stiffness and, at the same time, structural resistance to wind loads. Soma mentioned that the lamellas "… induce compression forces to create the complex elastic deformation. They reduce the distance between the two bearings and in this way induce a bending which results in a side rotation of the lamella" [46] (**Figure 13**).

Movement of the lamellas control light conditions in the foyer and the best practice area; in addition it creates animated patterns on the façade like ocean waves. These movements can also be likened to the gills of a fish [48].

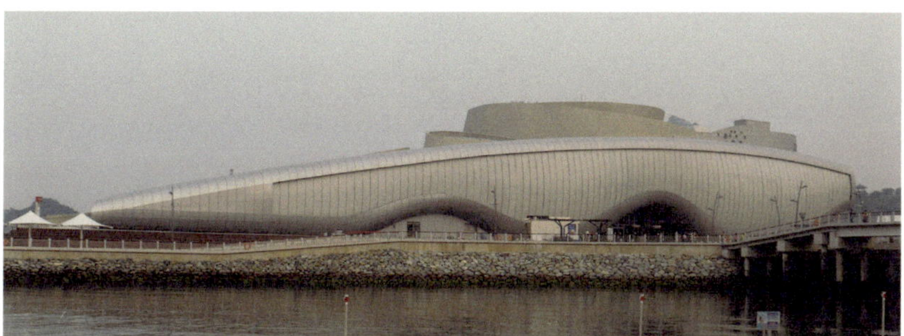

Figure 13. The kinetic façade and closed lamellas [47].

4.3. Smog-eating façades

Photocatalytic TiO_2 in the cement developed by Italcementi is known as smog-eating material for the last few years. Although it has been in use since 1995, the first patent had only a self-cleaning effect and was applied in many outstanding works, such as Misericordia Church in Rome or Cite de la Musique et des Beaux Arts, some tunnels or pavements, etc. "TX Active" technology, which was generated in 2006, added air cleaning property to the material [49]. The material captures air pollution when the façade comes into contact with light, then transforms the pollution to inert salts, and thus reduces smog levels in the environment. This new formulation was utilized in the two contemporary buildings, and their investigations are given as follows.

One of them is a façade design for Manuel Gea Gonzalez Hospital building in Mexico City, which is one of the most polluted megacities in the world. The original hospital building was constructed in 1942, and in 2013 a new building (named Torre de Especialidades) was added with a smog-eating façade [50]. The 2500 m^2 façade is designed by Berlin-based architecture firm Elegant Embellishments. TiO_2 can act as a catalyst for chemical reactions when it is activated by sunlight. When UV rays hit the tiles, a reaction occurs, converting mono-nitrogen oxides (the substances that make smog smoky) into less harmful substances such as calcium nitrate and water, along with some CO_2. The TiO_2 in the tiles does not wear; it can keep on doing photocatalysis indefinitely.

The tiles' irregular and biomimetic pattern is a quasicrystalline or Penrose grid based on sponges and corals and was designed by Prosolve through Rhino (**Figure 14**). Prosolve's modules are manufactured from an ABS-polycarbonate plastic sheet; it is vacuum-formed over aluminum tools, then cut, and coated by a robotic sprayer with layers of TiO_2 and primers that adhere to the plastic substrate. The reliefs increase the absorption surface and reduce the

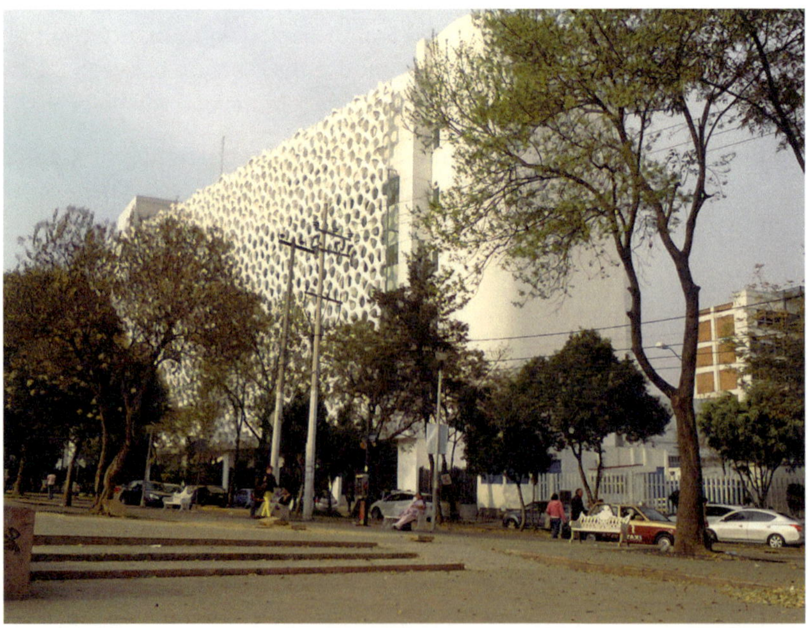

Figure 14. Façade of Torre de Especialidades [51].

speed of the wind, generating turbulences that better distribute the polluting particles over the surface of the cells. Since each piece of the puzzle has multiple reliefs, polluting particles can be captured from various directions [50]. The architects hope that the building can counteract the impact of air pollution and provide slightly fresher air into the hospital's immediate area. According to the developers, the façade will negate the effects of up to 1000 cars a day.

Expo 2015 Italian Pavilion was designed by an Italian architectural firm, Nemesi and Partners (**Figure 15**). The 13,000 m^2 building has six floors and presents Italy's past, present, and future through images, dynamic digital projections on mirrored walls, ceilings, and floors and accompanied by vibrant rhythms. The 9000 m^2 façade contains 900 biodynamic concrete panels. Around 80% of this air-purifying cement is made from recycled materials, such as scraps from Carrara marble. Italcementi tests have demonstrated that the photocatalytic cement can reduce NO_X levels from 20 to 80%, depending on atmospheric conditions. According to researches, the reduction of NO_X concentration calculated is around 45% in the area covered by the TX Active® blocks [49].

Nemesi and Partners wanted the building to act like a kind of urban jungle, not only esthetically but by also mimicking the role of trees in city landscapes—which naturally help purify the air. Inspired by nature, the final design resembles large stretched out tree branches which wrap themselves around the iconic building: "The overall concept of the architectural design of the Italian Pavilion is that of an urban forest in which the building, through its skin and its volumetric arrangement, takes on the features of an architectural landscape… The branching pattern of the external cladding of Palazzo Italia coherently interprets the theme of the tree of life, inserting it in the form of a petrified forest" [52].

4.4. Cultivating algae

Algae are cellular organisms that have been the precursors to plants, and they can make photosynthesis more efficiently than many plant species. In this context, they can remove CO_2 from their environments and produce O_2. Algae live in a hydrophilic environment and can be grown in photo-bioreactors on earth. The first application of photo-bioreactors in a building façade

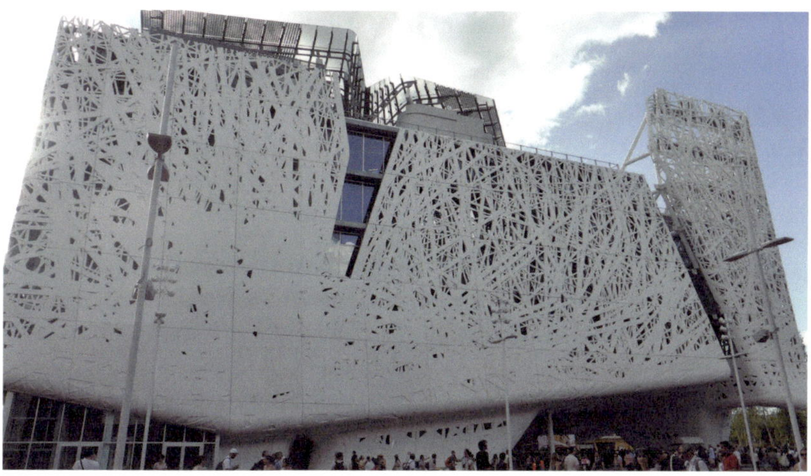

Figure 15. Facade of the Italian Pavilion in Expo 2015, by TBT, 2015.

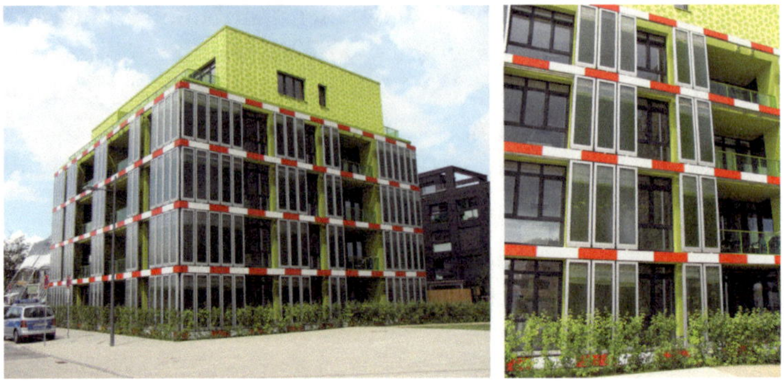

Figure 16. BIQ Apartment House: (left) exterior [53] and (right) closer view of panels [54].

is on BIQ apartment building (2013), designed by Splitterwerk and Graz and by engineering firm Arup in Hamburg, Germany. BIQ is a cubic, five-story building and is an abbreviation for "building with a Bio-Intelligent Quotient." It was constructed as a part of the International Building Exhibition of 2013 (**Figure 16**). The algae façade serves as a buffer between the indoors and the outdoors and supplies both thermal heating and biomass for the building.

The 200 m^2 façade contains 129 photo-bioreactor panels with 2.5 × 0.7 m dimensions. They were assembled on a secondary structure in front of the house façade. Flat plate photo-bioreactor panels were used on the façade because of their high transformative efficiency to receive UV light. The algae are continuously supplied with liquid nutrients and CO_2 via a water circuit running through the façade. The light rays are absorbed by the façade and generate heat the same way a solar thermal unit does, which is then either used directly for hot water and heating or stored in the ground using boreholes [55].

When algae are ready to be harvested, they are transferred as a thick pulp to the technical room inside the building and fermented in a biogas plant. The performance of the algae façade elements was measured for 1 year. For this year, the biomass production at the façade was on average 15 g/day and was stored alongside the biogas production machine. It also produced 30 kWh/m^2 biomass and 150 kWh/m^2 heat energy. Thus the annual CO_2 emission of the building was reduced by 6 tons [55].

In addition, this façade has an important interactive surface for city and should be considered with its aesthetical quality like Jan Wurm (Arup) said: "As well as generating renewable energy and providing shade to keep the inside of the building cooler on sunny days, it also creates a visually interesting look that architects and building owners will like" [56].

Köktürk et al. have proposed a diamond-shaped flat plate photobioreactor façade system [57]. They have also designed a monitor and management system for their façade. The temperature is kept at 37–38°C, and the heat released from the system is used for hot water or for air conditioning with a heat exchanger. Accordingly, these buildings were not only inspired from nature but also embodied it as a component.

5. Conclusion

Despite all the advances in technology and environment-centered debates, the environmental footprint of the human race and buildings continues to increase. This is mainly because of increasing population and increase in comfort requirements. Nature creates sustainable environments and surrounds us with answers to most of the questions about sustainability since it has worked for millennia to perfect solutions. This thinking has permeated among some designers. They take inspiration and learn from nature on the road to become more sustainable and having less environmental impact. The most common approach is formal and functional biomimicry; in façades, some building elements and materials are even called biomimetic. The concept of biomimicry is in harmony with the concept of sustainability; however, there are many degrees of sustainability, and each and every biomimetic application is not always sustainable. The sustainability principles should be at the core of the design problem definition and its unique design constraints to reach a sustainable future.

This chapter has provided examples to biomimetic design approaches in the context of three main aspects in designing a sustainable façade; energy requirements, form, and structure; and sustainability considerations. Another way to make use of and learn from nature in design is biodesign, a way of bio-cooperation with natural elements. Biodesign is a relatively new term, yet the approach has been around for centuries as traditional elements such as green walls. While there are various conceptual studies, biodesign has very few built examples apart from its traditional interpretation. One of the limiting factors in utilizing biodesign is its big scope that requires a multidisciplinary approach with input from diverse disciplines that are not usually involved in the construction sector, such as biologists and bioengineers. Biodesign works go beyond biomimicry and bring an innovative way to look at and work with nature; therefore, their applications will probably become more widespread in façade designs of the future.

Acknowledgements

Funginsulation is a product developed by Diploid. The authors would like to thank TBT and Diploid for the use of funginsulation in this work.

Author details

Ayça Tokuç[1]*, Fatma Feyzal Özkaban[1] and Özge Andiç Çakır[2]

*Address all correspondence to: ayca.tokuc@deu.edu.tr

1 Department of Architecture, Dokuz Eylül University, Izmir, Turkey

2 Department of Civil Engineering, Ege University, Izmir, Turkey

References

[1] Kuday I. Examination of the term biomimicry as a supporting factor indesign process [thesis]. Institute of Natural and Applied Sciences, Istanbul: Mimar Sinan Fine Arts University; 2009

[2] West M, Coar L. Biomimetic construction. In: Change Architecture Education Practices Proceedings of the 2012 ACSA International Conference; 20-22 June 2012; Barcelona, Spain; 2012. pp. 235-240

[3] Asefi M, Afzali Z. Environmentally sustainable architecture: Material-based technological design approach. Current World Environment. 2016;**11**(1):28

[4] Benyus JM. Biomimicry: Innovation Inspired by Nature. New York: Harper Perennial Publishing; 2002

[5] Aksamija A. Sustainable Façades: Design Methods for High-Performance Building Envelopes. New Jersey: Wiley; 2013

[6] Loonen RCGM. Bio-inspired adaptive building skins. In: Pacheco Torgal F, Labrincha JA, Diamanti MV, Yu CP, Lee HK, editors. Biotechnologies and Biomimetics for Civil Engineering. Cham: Springer International Publishing; 2015. pp. 115-134

[7] Craig S, Harrison D, Cripps A, Knott D. BioTRIZ suggests radiative cooling of buildings can be done passively by changing the structure of roof insulation to let longwave infrared pass. Journal of Bionic Engineering. 2008;**5**(1):55-66

[8] Dahl R. Cooling concepts: Alternatives to air conditioning for a warm world. Environmental Health Perspectives. 2013;**121**(1):a18

[9] Martín-Palma RJ, Lakhtakia A. Engineered biomimicry for harvesting solar energy: A bird's eye view. International Journal of Smart and Nano Materials. 2013;**4**(2):83-90

[10] Poppinga S, Zollfrank C, Prucker O, Rühe J, Menges A, Cheng T, Speck T. Toward a new generation of smart biomimetic actuators for architecture. Advanced Materials. 2017. DOI: 2017.10.1002/adma.201703653

[11] Szczyrba S. Human and nature symbiosis: Biomimic architecture as the paradigm shift in mitigation of impact on the environment [thesis]. Miami University; 2016

[12] Arslan S, Gönenç SA. Mimari Tasarım Paradigmasında Biomimesis'in Etkisi. Gazi Mimarlık Mühendislik Fakültesi Dergisi. 2007;**22**(2):451-460

[13] Gruber P, McGinley T, Muehlbauer M. Towards an agile biodigital architecture: Supporting a dynamic evolutionary and developmental view of architecture. In: Esteves AT, editor. 3rd International Conference of Biodigital Architecture and Genetics. 2017

[14] Tuğrul F, Savaşır K. Biyomimetik Mimarlık Kavramının Sürdürülebilirlik Bağlamında İrdelenmesi. In: Sürdürülebilir Yapı Tasarımı Konferansı. 2012

[15] Speck T, Knippers J, Speck O. Self-X materials and structures in nature and technology: Bioinspiration as a driving force for technical innovation. Architectural Design. 2015;**85**(5):34-39

[16] By Egdir (Own Work) [Public Domain], via Wikimedia Commons

[17] By Hamidreza (Own Work) [CC BY-SA 3.0 (https://creativecommons.org/licenses/by-sa/3.0)], via Wikimedia Commons

[18] Forouzanfar MH et al. Global, regional, and national comparative risk assessment of 79 behavioural, environmental and occupational, and metabolic risks or clusters of risks in 188 countries, 1990-2013: A systematic analysis for the Global Burden of Disease Study 2013. The Lancet. 2015;**386.10010**:2287-2323

[19] ch2 setting a new world standard in green building design. 2004. Melbourne City Council

[20] Badarnah L, Kadri U. A methodology for the generation of biomimetic design concepts. Architectural Science Review. 2015;**58**(2):120-133

[21] By Annette Teng [CC BY 3.0 (http://creativecommons.org/licenses/by/3.0)], via Wikimedia Commons

[22] Loonen RCGM, Trčka M, Cóstola D, Hensen JLM. Climate adaptive building shells: State-of-the-art and future challenges. Renewable and Sustainable Energy Reviews. 2013;**25**:483-493

[23] Ottelé M. A green building envelope: A crucial contribution to biophilic cities. In: Pacheco Torgal F, Labrincha JA, Diamanti MV, Yu CP, Lee HK, editors. Biotechnologies and Biomimetics for Civil Engineering. Cham: Springer International Publishing; 2015. pp. 135-161

[24] Bhushan B, Jung YC. Natural and biomimetic artificial surfaces for superhydrophobicity, self-cleaning, low adhesion, and drag reduction. Progress in Materials Science. 2011;**56**:1-108

[25] Gao H, Wang X, Yao H, Gorb S, Arzt E. Mechanics of hierarchical adhesion structures of geckos. Mechanics of Materials. 2005;**37**(2):275-285

[26] Gao X, Jiang L. Biophysics: Water-repellent legs of water striders. Nature. 2004;**432**(7013): 36-36

[27] Bechert DW, Bruse M, Hage W. Experiments with three-dimensional riblets as an idealized model of shark skin. Experiments in Fluids. 2000;**28**(5):403-412

[28] Fujishima A, Zhang X, Tryk D. TiO_2 photocatalysis and related surface phenomena. Surface Science Reports. 2008;**63**(12):515-582

[29] Burton A. Titanium dioxide photocleans polluted air. Environmental Health Perspectives. 2012;**120**(6):8043

[30] Boden SA, Bagnall DM. Bio-mimetic subwavelength surfaces for near-zero reflection sunrise to sunset. In: Photovoltaic Energy Conversion, Conference Record of the 2006 IEEE 4th World Conference on. IEEE. 2006. pp. 1358-1361

[31] Yang Q, Zhang Xa, Bagal A, Guo W, Chang C-H. Antireflection effects at nanostructured material interfaces and the suppression of thin-film interference. Nanotechnology. 2013;**24**(23):235202

[32] Soares N, Costa JJ, Gaspar AR, Santos Soares PN, et al. Review of passive PCM latent heat thermal energy storage systems towards buildings' energy efficiency. Energy and Buildings. 2013;**59**:82-103

[33] Tokuç A, Yesügey SC, Başaran T. An evaluation methodology proposal for building envelopes containing phase change materials: The case of a flat roof in Turkey's climate zones. Architectural Science Review. 2017;**60**(5):408-423

[34] Sardá C, Gómez Pioz J. Architectural bio-photo reactors: Harvesting microalgae on the surface of architecture. In: Pacheco Torgal F, Labrincha JA, Diamanti MV, Yu CP, Lee HK, editors. Biotechnologies and Biomimetics for Civil Engineering. Cham: Springer International Publishing. 2015. pp. 163-179

[35] Öncel SŞ, Köse A, Öncel DŞ. Façade integrated photobioreactors for building energy efficiency. In: Start-Up Creation. 2016. pp. 237-299

[36] Satyanarayana T, Prakash A, Johri BN. Microorganisms in environmental management: Microbes and environment. Microorganisms in Environmental Management: Microbes and Environment. 2012;**9789400722293**:1-819

[37] Van Breugel K. Is there a market for self-healing cement-based materials. In: Proc. First Int. Conf. Self Heal. Mater. 2007. pp. 1-9

[38] Madigan MT, Martinko JM, Stahl DA, Clark DP. 2000, Brock Biology of Microorganisms. 13th edition

[39] Cloud 9, Media-Tic Building Press Release [Internet]. 2007. Available from: https://slowlyturningimagery.files.wordpress.com/2015/08/presentacionmedia-tic_web_en.pdf [Accessed: 2017-12-12]

[40] By Zarateman (Own work) [CC0], via Wikimedia Commons

[41] Juaristi M, Monge-Barrio A. Adaptive façades in temperate climates. An in-use assessment of an office building. In: 11th Conference on Advanced Building Skins. 2016

[42] Google maps [Internet]. 2018. Available from: http://maps.google.com, Imagery ©2018 SKEnergy [Accessed: 2018-01-18]

[43] Composites and architecture [Internet]. 2012. Available from: http://compositesandarchitecture.com/?p=68 [Accessed: 2018-01-14]

[44] Masselter T, Poppinga S, Lienhard J, Schleicher S, Knippers J, Speck T. The flower of Strelitzia reginae as concept generator for the development of a technical deformation system for architectural purposes. In: 7th Plant Biomechanics International Conference—Clermont-Ferrand, August 2012. p. 391

[45] From Bermuda Botanical Gardens taken by Lauren Chickadel on June 28th, 2006. Strelitzia reginae

[46] In Progress: One Ocean/soma [Internet]. 2012. Available from: https://www.archdaily.com/208700/in-progress-one-ocean-soma [Accessed: 2017-12-15]

[47] By hyolee2 (Own work) [CC BY-SA 3.0 (https://creativecommons.org/licenses/by-sa/3.0) or GFDL (http://www.gnu.org/copyleft/fdl.html)], via Wikimedia Commons

[48] James M. FAÇADE-Integrated Sustainable Technologies for Tall Buildings: A discussion of the extent of adoption of such technologies in the most sustainable fifth generation tall buildings and the trends of the future. International Journal of Engineering Technology, Management and Applied Sciences. 2017;**5**(5)

[49] Topličić-Ćurčić G, Jevtić D, Grdić D, Ristić N, Grdić Z. Photocatalytic concrete—Environment friendly material. In: 5th International Conference Contemporary Achievements in Civil Engineering 21; April 2017; Subotica, Serbia

[50] Salla F. Rhino projects: A smog-eating façade [Internet]. 2014. Available from: http://blog.visualarq.com/2014/03/07/rhino-projects-a-smog-eating-façade/ [Accessed: 2018-01-17]

[51] By ArCaRa [CC BY 3.0 (http://creativecommons.org/licenses/by/3.0)], via Wikimedia Commons

[52] Palazzo Italia to get air-purifying facade for Milan Expo 2015 [Internet]. 2014. Available from: https://newatlas.com/palazzo-italia-milan-expo-smog-purifying-facade/32204/ [Accessed: 2017-12-12]

[53] By NordNordWest, Lizenz: Creative Commons by-sa-3.0 de [CCFoto: NordNordWest]

[54] By Lizenz: Creative Commons by-sa-3.0 de [CC BY-SA 3.0 de (https://creativecommons.org/licenses/by-sa/3.0/de/deed.en)], via Wikimedia Commons

[55] Wurm J. The bio-responsive façade. Detail Green. 2013;**1**:62-65

[56] Chalcraft E. Arup Unveils World's First Algae-powered Building [Internet]. 2013. Available from: https://www.dezeen.com/2013/04/15/arup-unveils-worldsfirst-algae-powered-building/. [Accessed: 2017-11-14]

[57] Köktürk G, Ünal A, Tokuç A. A new approach for a control system of an innovative building-integrated photobioreactor. In: Exergetic, Energetic and Environmental Dimensions. London: Academic Press; pp. 71-85

Chapter 6

Bio-Inspired Adaptable Façade Control Reflecting User's Behavior

Hyunsoo Lee and Nayeon Kim

Additional information is available at the end of the chapter

http://dx.doi.org/10.5772/intechopen.72917

Abstract

The purpose of this research is to develop the process of methodology in designing adaptable façade. This study focuses on the processes of façade operation control for each resident's unit according to the user's lifestyle. This study aims to develop the design methods that are applicable to the adaptable facade, which is inspired by the design inspiration of the biomimicry. The ideal façade to increase comfort in internal space is an adaptable façade that can constantly respond to changes in the environments. This chapter attempts in active adoption of adaptable facade that makes it possible to respond to changing requirements and environments, eventually enabling the creation of customized services for users. This chapter explores the processes of designing an adaptable façade controlled by three rules inspired by the behaviors of flocks of birds. This chapter shows how adopted bird intelligence can produce various façade controls. Also, this chapter demonstrates biomimetic façade control that has been implemented by behavior-based design. Through this demonstration, this chapter identifies the potentials of biomimetic design in facade using rules of bird flocking as source of design inspiration. This study concludes that a behavior-based approach provides flexibly responding façade to environments increasing users' quality of life.

Keywords: biomimicry, adaptable facade, responsive architecture, behavior-oriented design, kinetic façade, façade control, bird flocking

1. Introduction

What is a façade? A façade is generally one exterior side of a building, usually the front, and the word comes from the French *façade*, which means "face." In architecture, the façade remains, from a design perspective, the most important aspect of a building. It is an essential architectural element, because a building's façade determines the initial impression that a building makes. In addition to the role it plays with regard to esthetic design, the building façade also serves to divide external and internal space and plays an important role in interacting with the outside environment. However, the environment is constantly changing. In arts, Monet painted a series of expressions of the ever-changing world. Monet painted images that change over time. This is the reason why Monet painted his *Rouen Cathedral* series more than 30 times, always at different times of the day and year. The series reflects many views of the same subject under different lighting conditions. Through this artwork, Monet would have wanted to prove that constant change is the truth of the world. In this regard, a good building must be capable of changing itself by accepting and responding constant variations in the environment [1, 13, 14].

In the ever-changing environment, the architectural façade should have functional performances to protect human beings inside. The external environment changes continuously. One of the architectural elements to meet the functions is a facade. When designing the façade, architects need to consider external factors such as natural sunlight, temperature, humidity, precipitation, wind, and earthquake. The façade protects people by creating a boundary between the inside and the outside. It is also important because it provides thermal comfort. For example, the façade of *Notre dame du Haut*, a Catholic chapel in Ronchamp, France, built in 1954, presents a picturesque image and also helps to fulfill peoples' psychological needs by allowing a generous amount of natural light to reach those inside the thermal insulation of the external wall, saving energy as well providing a comfortable environment. However, this building has limitations: the curtain walls of the building are fixed, and it cannot respond flexibly to the fluctuating environment. We believe that the ultimate façade should be able to respond adaptably to the ever-changing environment. Although the ideal is that a building should respond to changes in the environment like a living creature, most buildings are not satisfactory in this regard. For example, one of the most representative modern buildings is *Lake Shore Drive Apartments* in Chicago, designed by Mies Van Der Rohe. This skyscraper exhibits both the spirit of the twentieth century machine esthetic and minimalism; the building has no decorative elements and is simply made of glass with metal structures. However, a weakness of this building's façade is that it seems very static, and there is no user control of the façade. That is, it is impossible for residents to control the function of the façade at the level of the individual apartment unit. The building offers spectacular views to residents through transparent glass, but the level of thermal comfort is not optimal. In other words, fixed windows that cannot open and close have reduced the building's ability to respond to the environment.

An ideal facade must be able to respond to changes in the environment [18]. An adaptable façade does this, and since it can extend the life of a building, it contributes to the development of sustainable architecture [21]. An adaptable façade is able to interact with natural adaptive systems in order to respond continuously to the environment [9]. Typically, these buildings efficiently utilize windows in order to optimize façade illumination and building performance by interacting with the environment [8]. The drawback of previously built façades is that they do not provide people with the ability to control the environment [10]. Most buildings focus primarily on performance-oriented design rather than user-oriented design. Previous studies have emphasized technical, performance-based facade design, and it is difficult to find adaptable façades that respond to users' lifestyles and behaviors. Many architects have difficulty in designing façades that are responsive to users' various lifestyle requirements and in incorporating these into façade design [5]. The building façade should have features to optimize environmental performance as well as to consider the esthetic of building. The façade, in particular, should take into consideration the user's individual lifestyle and preference [19]. In order to overcome the limitations of existing buildings, this study explores user-oriented façade design.

The main purpose of this research is to develop a methodology for designing adaptable façades. This study focuses on the processes of façade operation control for each resident's unit, allowing the user to adjust the façade to match the user's lifestyle. This study aims to develop a design method inspired by the concept of biomimicry that is applicable to the development of adaptable facades. The study's first objective is to propose applicable methods of façade design based on an interpretation of the rules of bird flocking. The second objective is to develop a design process that can be applied to a façade's louver controls. The last objective is to develop an application example and identify the potential of the design process developed by this study.

2. Theoretical background

2.1. Adjustable façades and adaptable façades

The concept of adaptation in architecture aims to increase the usability of building functions in response to the external environment or the user's behavior [22]. In other words, adaptable architecture results in sustainable buildings with extended lifespans by allowing buildings to make flexible changes to adapt to changing exterior environments [21]. The positive consequences of using methods to design adaptable façades include extending the lifespan of the building as well as improving the quality of human life. Designing adaptable façades not only prolongs the lives of buildings that use them but also improves the quality of human life. In this chapter, the types of adaptable façade design are divided into two types: adjustable façades and adaptable façades. To provide people with the ability to control the environment, we must plan for an adjustable façade. In an adjustable façade, the user can open and close the window or rotate the louvers to respond to the environment. It is a façade type that has been in existence for a long time and users manually control it. Adjustable façades allow for the manipulation of architectural elements by, for example, opening or closing windows and changing the angle of a louver.

An adaptable façade is a façade that can automatically adjust the environment using technology, whereas an adjustable façade provides the user with manual control over the environment. An adaptable façade differs from a traditional façade; in that it incorporates adjustable devices whose capacity for interactive control enables the building envelope to act as a climate moderator. By using the façade in this way, we can provide a building with the ability to accept or reject free energy from the external environment and, as a result, to reduce the amount of artificial energy required to achieve comfortable internal conditions. One notable example of an adaptable façade is *Al Bahr Tower*, located in Abu Dhabi. Al Bahr Tower designed by AHR studio has the world's largest dynamic façade, and this adaptive shading system of façade is designed to detect changes in the climate and save energy. The other building examples include *One Ocean EXPO pavilion* in Yeosou, Korea, *Syddansk Universitet* communications and design building in Kolding, Denmark, and *Media-TIC* building in Barcelona, Spain [12]. The façade of *One Ocean* EXPO pavilion 2012 by SOMA architect consists of 108 kinetic fins as the opening elements. These fins called lamellas are reinforced at the top and bottom edges of the façade and provide a high tensile strength as well as a low bending firmness. The advantage of this facade enables large reversible elastic deformations [24]. In case of *Syddansk Universitet* building designed by Henning Larsen architect, it has a sustainable feature in a climate-responsive kinetic facade that adjusts to the changing daylight and controls interior temperatures for occupants. The Media-TIC building designed by architects Cloud 9 is also a good example of an adaptable façade. Using technology of sensor monitoring including occupancy, light, temperature, and humanity as well as renewable energy generation, it consequently creates a near net zero energy in building [23].

Adaptable architecture offers an optimal environment for users inside. The façade is able to interact with natural adaptive systems to respond constantly to changes in the environment [9]. Typically, these buildings utilize windows efficiently to optimize façade illumination and to optimize building performance by interacting with the environment [8]. However, the problem with this façade is that it does not provide sufficient user control. Although adaptable building envelopes have positive aspects in achieving internal comfort for occupants and building energy efficiency, it still needs much more exploration in social and cultural aspects [12].

2.2. Façade design method using biomimicry

Principles of nature such as sustainability, bio-architecture, biophilia, biomimicry, and biomimetic architecture can help to address the environmental crisis of contemporary architecture and to provide more comfortable user spaces. Biomimetic architecture, which is the focus of this chapter, is a modern architectural philosophy that seeks to find solutions to architectural design challenges presented by every day changes in the environment around a given building [11, 15]. Biomimicry is not only a rapidly growing design principle in engineering, but it is also emerging as an important architectural principle. Problem solving by biomimicry is an approach that makes use of principles, mechanisms, and strategies found in nature [3, 4]. Janine Benyus, a pioneer in biomedical research in the United States, introduced the concept of biomimicry in 1997. Biomimicry is a concept that is inspired by nature, exploring sustainable solutions and applying them to design. The word is a combination of two Greek roots: *bios,* which means life, and mimesis, which means mimicry or imitation [23]. A typical example of an environmentally functional facade system utilizing a biomimicry design motif is the *Arab World Institute* designed by Jean Nouvel. The facade of the building measures and compares the luminance of the outside environment with the luminance inside the building and then adjusts the luminance using a window opening and closing device, providing an optimal illumination environment inside the building [17].

However, although this performance-based approach provides beneficial features for controlling facades, it is not feasible to satisfy all residents' individual needs or requirements of viable environmental performance. This is because it provides a standardized performance without considering individual preferences. Another limitation with the performance-based approach is that it did not take into account the psychological needs of residents. People do not always have the same demands and the degree of demand varies according to the change of mood and situation.

http://dx.doi.org/10.5772/intechopen.72917

This performance-based approach seeks for optimization to meet the building efficiency, but the optimized outcome might not be ideal for residents. In order to solve these drawbacks, this chapter proposes a behavior-based approach rather than performance-based approach. It is assumed that the control of the facade according to occupant behaviors such as lifestyles is more advantageous in terms of psychological and environmentally sustainable aspect for occupants. As a strategy to get inspiration for this behavior-based approach, the theory of the biomimicry is adopted. The biomimicry approach can improve the quality of the facade design by developing the facade control method based on the self-organization and collective behavior of the community [16]. In this study, as biomimicry approach, swarm intelligence theory is utilized. Terminology "swarm" has been wisely used to many areas including biology, engineering, computation and others. Swarm intelligence is firstly introduced by Beni and Wang, and it means the collective behaviors of self-organized system [2]. The collective behaviors include examples of army ants, bird flocking, animal herding, fish schooling, and collective swarms of bacteria and locusts [7]. Mainly, this study is focused on bird flocking behaviors.

3. Behavior-oriented adaptable façade

Based on the above background information, this research aims to develop a behavior-based adaptable façade. First, a set of rules inspired by the flying behaviors of flocking birds are established to apply to adaptable façade control. A set of rules of façade control were developed accordingly. By examining the application of the rules of façade control, this research is to verify and demonstrate the potential use of the behavior-oriented façade control system. There are three research components that we have chosen in order to resolve the façade design problem. To produce an adaptable façade, a bio-inspired design approach is adopted, using bird flocking intelligence [2], as our source of inspiration. The purpose of this research is to develop a façade control method that takes into account user behaviors.

In this study, three rules governing the flying behavior of birds inspire the control of the façade's louver. The first rule is that birds fly close to and in the same direction as neighboring birds. As shown in **Figure 1**, each bird follows the behavior of neighboring birds. It is an important goal of this study to attempt to adapt such traits to the behavior of residents in the

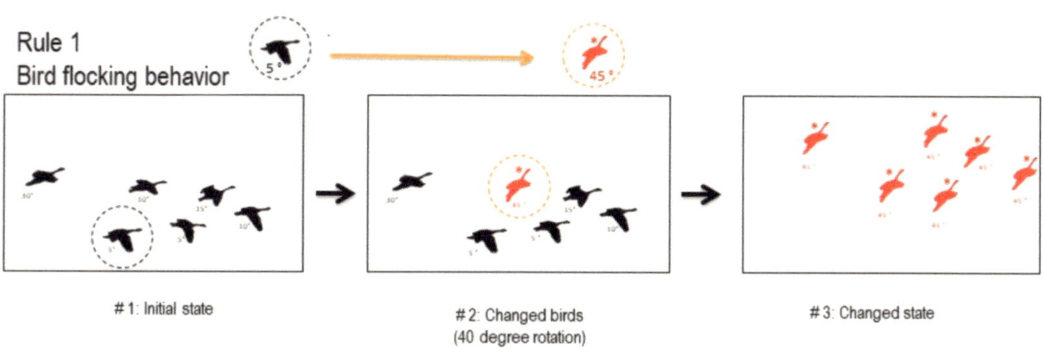

Figure 1. Rule 1: Adjacent birds react to each other in the same direction.

building. For example, if a person closes a window when it is raining heavily to prevent rain from entering the room, other people will tend to follow this person and close their windows as well. If a person is away and is not able to close the window by himself, it would be useful to set up a system that closes windows automatically when it is raining.

The second rule is that birds maintain a constant distance from neighboring birds when flying. Birds maintain regular intervals with their neighbors to avoid the collision. **Figure 2** is an example of the application of these laws. If a bird rotates by an angle of 30°, the rest of the birds can be interpreted as increasing its angle by 30° from its present angle. This principle can be used to increase the angle of each louver in the façade by 30° relative to the current louver angle.

The first and second rules described above might be too simple. We can apply more complex rules, but the complexity or simplicity of the rules applied is not important. The emphasis in this study is on architecturally interpreting the laws of bird behavior and thereby showing that the principles of these behaviors can be applied to architectural facades. However, an example of more complicated application method could explain the potential for the behavioral principle of birds. The third rule was developed with this perspective.

The last rule is to fly toward the central gravity in the groups of the same neighbors. As shown in **Figure 3**, birds tend to fly as groups. From this, it is possible to set the assumption that the same group behaves in the same way. Thus, if a group of members cause a change in behavior, birds in the other groups do not respond to the behavior, but it can be assumed that birds in the same group follow the same behavior. It can be considered that these subgroups exhibit the same behavior in some way similar to the first rule. However, the difference from the first rule is that it applies only to the group, not to the whole. These groups can be defined by the bird's flight, but they can be grouped into small groups according to lifestyle, age, and gender in a way that defines people. The characteristics of these residents are called residents' profiles in this study.

The last rule is to fly toward the central gravity in the groups of the same neighbors. As shown in **Figure 3**, birds tend to fly in groups. From this, it is possible to make the assumption that the same group behaves in the same way. Thus, if members of a given group change their behavior, birds in other groups will not respond to that change. However, it can be assumed

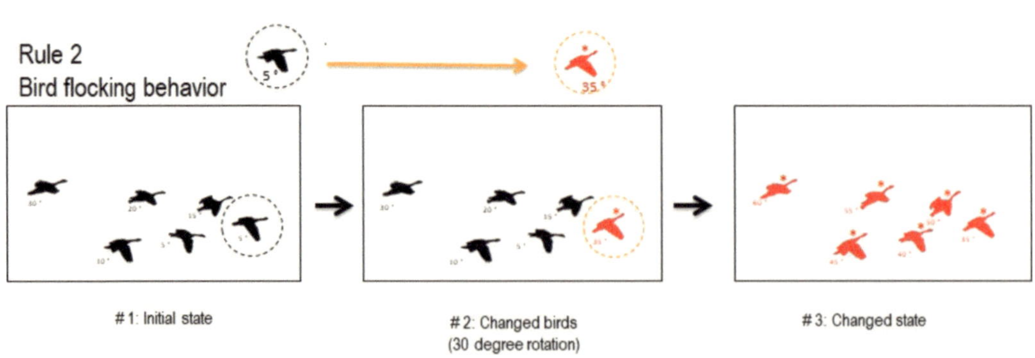

Figure 2. Rule 2: Birds' behavior keeping certain degree of flying angle.

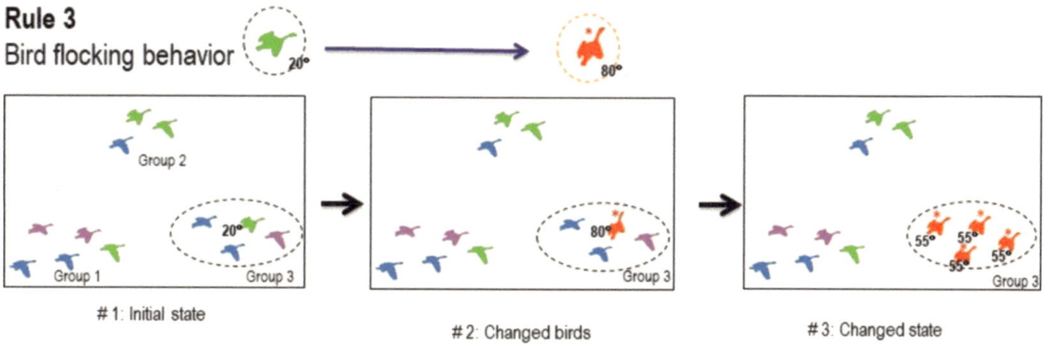

Figure 3. Rule 3: Birds' behavior to steer together average "center of gravity" of birds' group.

that behavior will change within a given group in response to changed behavior by one of birds. Thus, these subgroups appear to exhibit the same behavior, as in the first rule. However, the third rule differs from the first rule, and in that it applies only to the subgroups and not to the flock as a whole. These groups can be defined not only according to the birds' flight patterns, but also can be grouped into subgroups according to lifestyle, age, and gender, similar to human subgroups. In this study, these characteristics that define resident subgroups are called residents' profiles.

In this study, a case study was conducted to derive ideas about how to apply the three rules of bird flocking intelligence described above to façade control. As described above, we interpreted the birds' flying behavior and applied what we learned to the façade's louver control system. In other words, bird flocking behaviors were used as a source of inspiration for the creation of an adaptable façade corresponding to user's behaviors and lifestyles.

4. Bird flocking behavior-based adaptable façade design

Generally, architects or designers do not create designs in the absence of any reasons or inspirations. Many designs are inspired by something specific, and this is equally true for the design of architectural façades [25]. There are many things that inspire designers when designing a facade, but nature, in particular, is a frequent source of inspiration. In this respect, the biomimicry approach is very appropriate. In this chapter, we included two approaches to the design of an adaptable façade: a morphological design approach and a behavior-based design approach. **Figure 4** shows the morphological approach to biomimetic design described above. A morphological biomimetic design approach follows the form of life. In this example, a bird's profile and form are applied to an architectural façade. This method is straightforward and simple and therefore can be used easily by the designer. However, although this method has the advantage of providing a basis for façade design, it is not an effective example of using biomimicry.

Biomimicry design can be used to greater advantage by applying behavioral rules or rules inherent in living things rather than by applying such morphological methods. In this sense, the focus of this study is the behavior-based design approach. In this study, we propose a

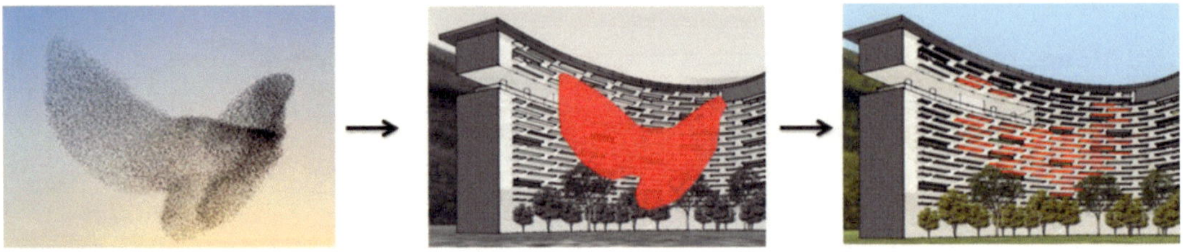

Figure 4. Morphological design approach: façade design inspired by bird flocking.

methodology of façade design based on bird flying behavior. We also conducted research on the assumption that behavior-based design controls are more effective than performance-based design controls. Most previous papers on façade design have adopted a performance-based design approach. However, the performance-based facade control is based on general services rather than on one-to-one custom services. As a solution to this problem, this study proposes a behavior-based design control method.

4.1. Façade control system

As shown in **Figure 5**, this study argues that residents' satisfaction can be improved by controlling the physical environment individually based on the occupant's behavior [25]. Our approach is to mimic the process of bird flocking and we developed control process of behavior-based physical environment. The idea is to interpret the behavior of the birds and create an adaptable façade that responds to the behavior of residents. Life-log data on residents' rules of behaviors in the building are the basis for making important decisions about controlling the physical environment. In developing such rules, we reinterpreted the behavior rules of birds and apply them to façade control. As shown in the figure, it is a process to control the façade louver based on using the user's life-log to control the physical environment. In this behavior-based facade control, the residents' life-log data play an important role.

As shown in **Figure 5**, this study argues that residents' satisfaction can be improved by controlling the physical environment individually based on the occupant's behavior. Our approach is to mimic the behaviors of flocking birds, and we developed a behavior-based process of controlling the physical environment. The idea is to interpret the behavior of the birds and to create an adaptable façade that responds to the behavior of residents. Life-log data on residents' rules of behavior in the building are the basis for making important decisions about how to control the physical environment. In developing such rules, we reinterpreted the behavior rules of birds and applied them to the façade control system. In this behavior-based facade control method, the residents' lifelog data play an important role to change the facade's louver.

4.2. Principle of facade application of birds' flocking pattern

In this study, we applied the three rules of bird flocking to the design of the façade pattern. **Table 1** shows the bird behavior-based rules applied to the facade louver controls. As shown in the table, the principles of bird flocking behavior are applied to the façade louver controls.

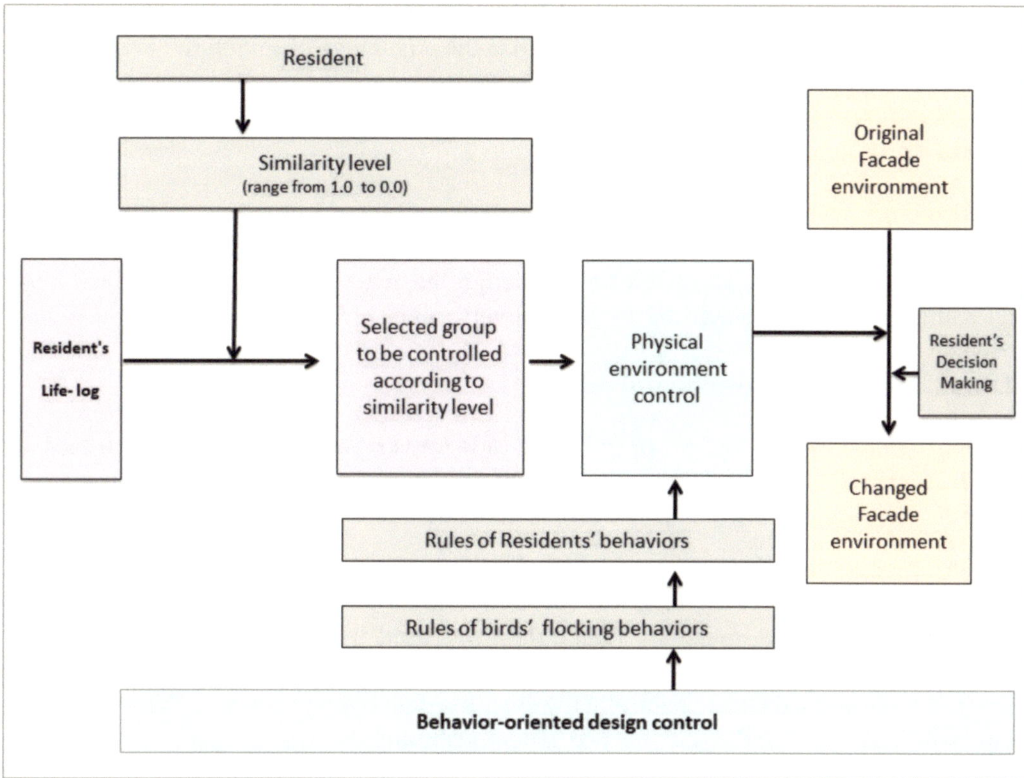

Figure 5. Control process of behavior-based physical environment.

	Bird flocking behaviors	Façade application
Rule 1	To align with same direction of bird's neighbor	To align with certain degree of louver
Rule 2	To keep certain degree of flying angles	To change certain degrees to adjacent louvers
Rule 3	To steer together average "center of gravity" of birds' group	To steer toward the "average of degree" of same group

Table 1. Bird flocking behavior and façade application.

5. Façade design process using bird flight rules

In this study, we will explain various methods of applying bird flight patterns to adaptable façades. We also developed a bird flight-inspired example of the process of finding design rules and applying them to façades. Through these applications, we have explained that principles of animal behavior can be used as a source of inspiration for biomimetic facades. This biomimetic façade design provides a systematic design framework for façades that responds to the user's lifestyle and preferences [9, 17]. Therefore, in this chapter, we prove that integrating design with the biological processes has the advantage of giving the architect more abundant design inspirations.

5.1. Case study

In this study, a *Lotte Buyeo Resort* building in the Republic of Korea was selected as a case study in order to apply the principles of bird flight to façade control. As shown in **Figure 6**, this façade has dozens of façade louvers. Although the actual building cannot adjust louver angles, this study assumes that the angle of louvers can be individually adjusted.

5.2. Residents' facade louver control data

In order to demonstrate how to control the facade louver, we have matched each bird and each facade louver corresponding to individual residents. The concept diagram is shown in **Figure 7**. This diagram is based on the lifelog data illustrated in **Figure 5**.

In order to create the behavior-based facade louver control proposed in this study [26], it is firstly necessary to collect the residents' behavioral data to control the angle of the facade louver. In this study, an imaginary lifelog data was used which is revised data of 24-hour self-diary to survey 53 residents in Korea [20]. Data collection of lifelog is a crucial research issue in behavior-based facade control. However, the data collection in this chapter is not the scope of the research. For the convenience of demonstrating the concept of the behavior-based facade control, an imaginary lifelog data is used. In this regard, **Figure 8**, which is revised and obtained based on the previous research [6], shows an illustrative example of how the louver of the facade is controlled based on the lifelog data. As shown in the figure, when the sensor detects illumination of daylighting, residents can make final decisions related to control on the facade using generalized behavior pattern. Behavior patterns include angle data of façade louver control made by residents. As shown in **Figure 8**, lifelog data may be accumulated by sensor technology. In future studies, based on the IOT, data collection for lifelog data needs to be further discussed.

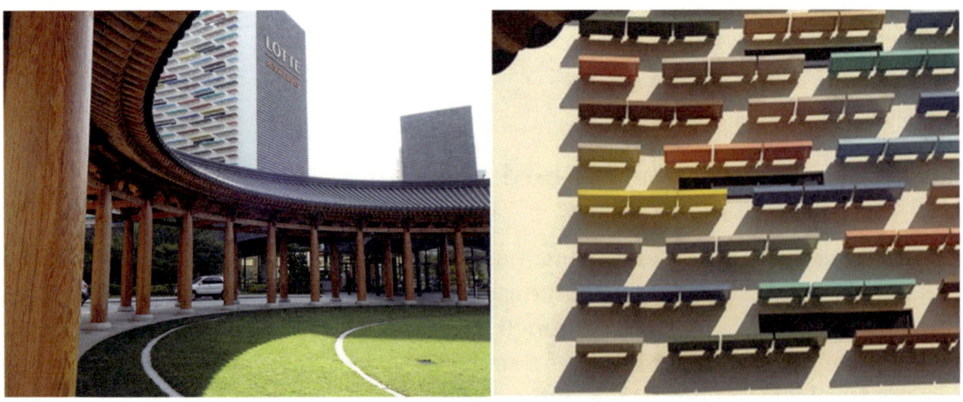

Figure 6. Buyeo Resort building, Republic of Korea.

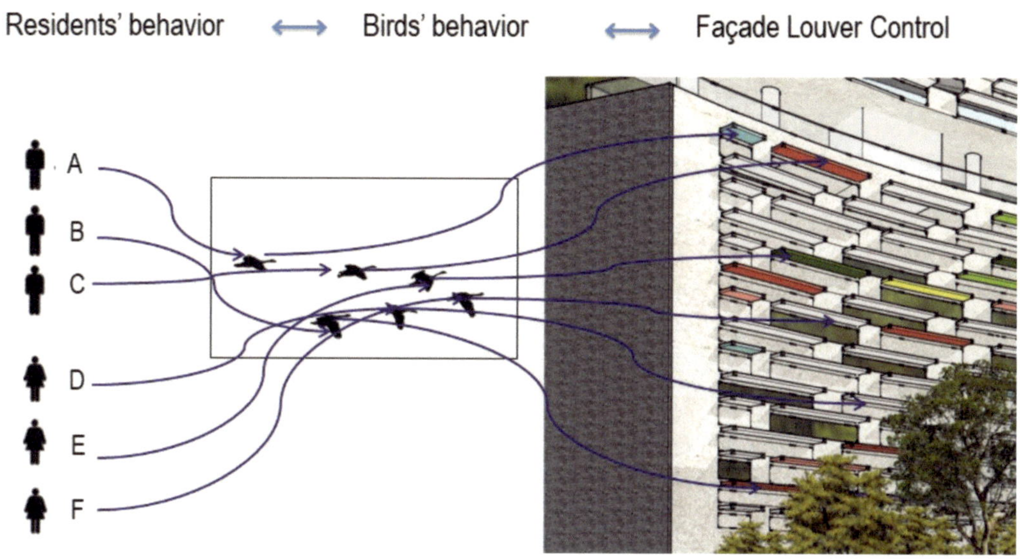

Figure 7. Conceptual diagram of residents' façade louver control.

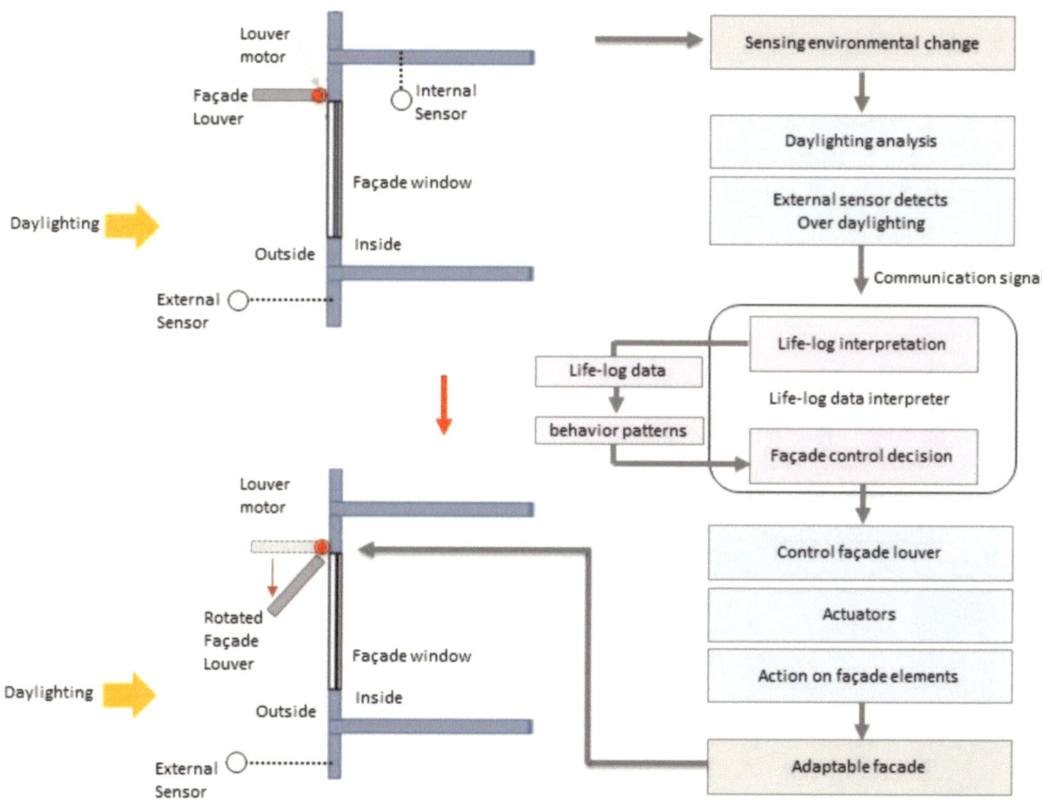

Figure 8. Diagram of sensor technology based façade operation system (modified from "Intelligent Envelopes for high-performance buildings" by [6]).

Figure 9 shows an example of collected data of the residents' previous behaviors pertaining to the façade louver angle. The lifelog is a record of user behavior. I argue that we should embed this behavioral data into a behavior-based adaptable façade design. After collecting previous lifelog data on the louver control angles used by the residents, we analyzed the residents who have similar behaviors based on this data.

Figure 10 is an example of data showing similar behavior among residents. For example, a similarity of 1.0 indicates the most identical behavior, and a similarity of 0.0 means that there is no identical behavior. The similarity of behavior is used to set the group of louvers to be controlled. The lower the similarity of behavior, the greater the number of louvers to be controlled. We created this similarity index in order to establish a basis for controlling the angles of louvers on a group-by-group basis.

The residents' façade louver control system determines whether louver control is required by sending a message to residents who show similar behavior, as shown in **Figure 11**, and asking them to make a decision. The reason to ask for the final decision on whether or not to change louver angle is that this individual user-oriented control is as important as group basis control. Although the system is pursuing automatic control on a group-by-group-basis, the ultimate goal is that the individual user eventually is able to decide that angles of louver in case of needs to change louver's angle.

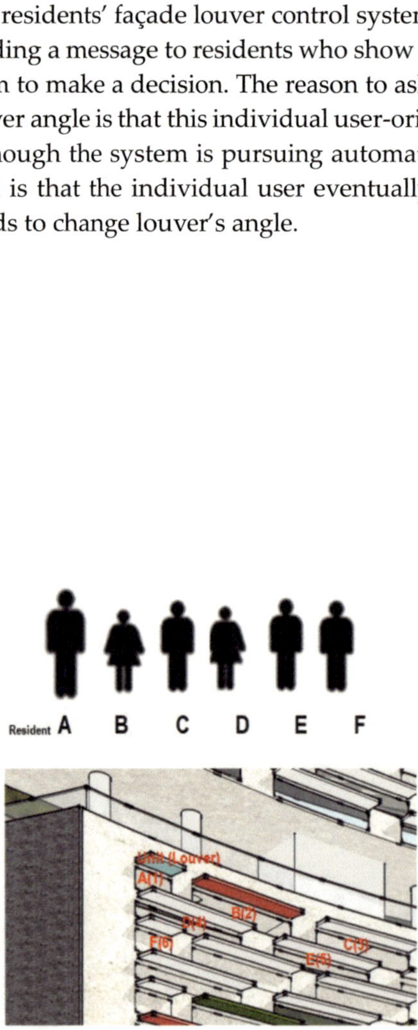

Resident	Residence Unit	Time	Façade Louver #	Louver Angle
A	1	7:00	1	30 degree
	1	12:00	1	90 degree
	1	17:00	1	45 degree
	1	21:00	1	- 45 degree
B	2	7:00	2	70 degree
	2	12:00	2	80 degree
	2	17:00	2	- 45 degree
	2	21:00	2	- 35 degree
C	3	7:00	3	90 degree
	3	12:00	3	70 degree
	3	17:00	3	- 15 degree
	3	21:00	3	48 degree
D	4	7:00	4	60 degree
	4	12:00	4	90 degree
	4	17:00	4	- 45 degree
	4	21:00	4	45 degree
E	5	7:00	5	50 degree
	5	12:00	5	85 degree
	5	17:00	5	- 35 degree
	5	21:00	5	40 degree
F	6	7:00	6	55 degree
	6	12:00	6	90 degree
	6	17:00	6	- 55 degree
	6	21:00	6	45 degree

Figure 9. Residents' behavior data collection.

❖ Level of similarity in Behaviors: Highest= 1.0 , Lowest =0.0

Resident	A	B	C	D	E	F	G	H	I	J	K	L	M	N	O
A	1.0	0.5	0.4	1.0	0.2	0.5	0.8	1.0	0.9	1.0	0.8	0.7	0.3	0.2	0.1
B			0.8	0.9	0.3	0.9	0.2	0.8	0.5	0.2	0.9	0.5	0.7	0.4	0.4
C				0.7	0.9	1.0	0.3	0.7	0.2	0.5	0.2	0.9	1.0	0.5	0.7
D					1.0	0.4	0.9	0.9	0.3	1.0	0.3	1.0	1.0	0.9	0.9
E						0.1	0.7	0.1	1.0	1.0	0.9	0.8	0.8	1.0	0.1
F							0.6	0.2	0.2	0.8	0.2	0.7	0.7	0.8	0.2
G								0.8	0.7	0.7	0.3	1.0	0.2	0.5	0.3
H									0.6	0.3	0.9	0.2	0.3	0.6	0.9
I										0.5	1.0	0.3	0.9	0.4	1.0
J											0.8	0.9	0.8	0.9	0.8
K												0.7	0.7	0.9	0.7
L													0.6	1.0	1.0
M														0.7	0.9
N															0.3
O															

Figure 10. Similarity level in behaviors between residents.

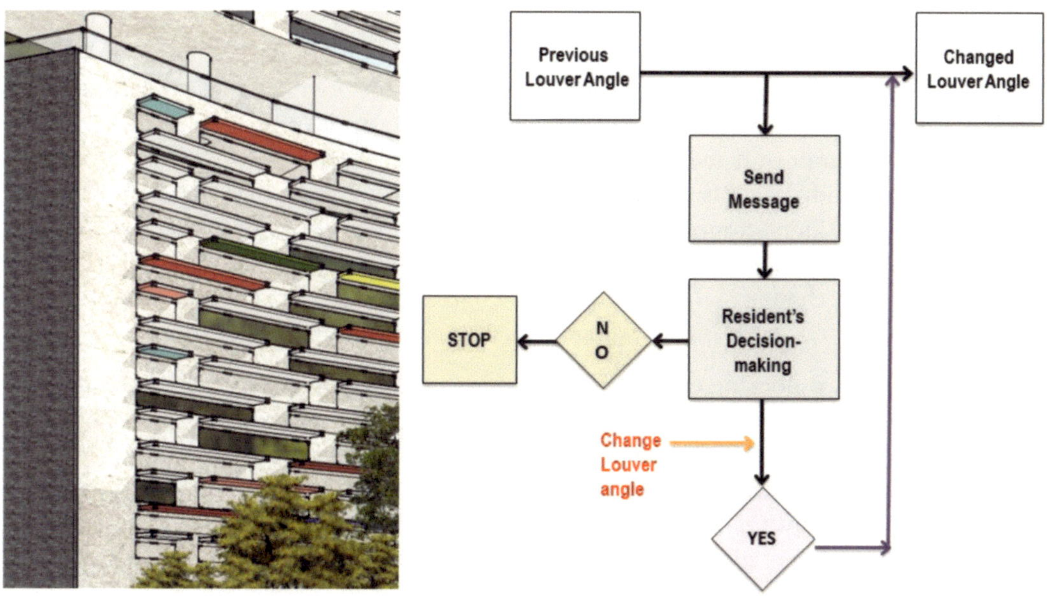

Figure 11. Façade louver control process by user's decision-making.

5.3. Behavior-based façade application

The first rule of bird flocking is that flocking birds align with a certain angle of flying. We interpreted this rule to mean that birds have a tendency to keep flying at an angle of the same degree. The first application example is shown in **Figure 12**. As shown in the figure, when the angle of one louver changes, the angle of another louver also changes to the same angle. This is an application of the principle described above that if one bird changes direction, the adjacent birds change direction, and the other birds change directions as they see the adjacent birds again. For facade applications, residents (A, E, J, L, and M) in a similar behavior pattern group also rotate 45° in the same direction if resident D changes the angle of the louver from 5 to 45°. In other words, all louvers of the same group will be changed to 45°, following the resident D. There is room for further study on the merit of the application of this principle in architectural performance. One of the advantages of applying these rules is that it creates a ripple effect through an entire group using one smart control. Currently, this represents only the beginning of the possibilities for control; this method will become more effective if it is refined by more advanced research on how to use it.

The bird flocking's rule 2 is that bird flocking keeps certain distance between birds to avoid collisions. Rule 2 interpreted in this chapter is that birds have a tendency to change flying with the angle of certain degree. The second rule is to control the facade louver by means of a bird's flight principle, which uniformly increases a certain angle of all current louver angles. As shown in **Figure 13**, if resident B rotates the louver angle by 30°, resident group (C, D, F, G, K) with similar behavior patterns also adjusts the angle by adding 30° from his angle. Therefore, each louver angle of user C, D, E, F, G, and K in group can be changed into 60, 50, 40, 35, and 45°. It is a principle that maintains a certain angle like keeping a certain distance of a bird.

The second rule of bird flocking described above is that flocking birds maintain a certain distance among themselves to avoid collisions. We interpret this to mean that birds have a tendency to change flying with the angle of certain degree. We applied this rule to the control of façade louvers by uniformly increasing or decreasing louver angles in a group in response to changes in an individual louver angle. As shown in **Figure 13**, if resident B increases the louver angle by 30°, the resident group (C, D, F, G, and K) with similar behavior patterns also adjusts the angle by adding 30° from his angle. Therefore, the louver angles user C, D, E, F, G, and K could, for example, change to 60, 50, 40, 35, and 45°, respectively. The principle is to maintain a certain angle the way birds in a flock maintain a certain distance among themselves.

The third rule of bird flocking is that flocking birds steer toward the average "center of gravity" of a given group of birds. We interpreted this rule to mean that birds have a tendency to keep flying at the same average angle. It is assumed that there are three groups of birds and only birds in group 3 have changed the angle from 20 to 80°. Then, whole birds in group 3 change flying degree into 55°. As indicated in **Figure 14**, if A changes the louver angle from 20 to 80°, the mean louver angle of residents A, D, H, and J is 55°. Therefore, the louver angles of unit A, D, H, and J in same group can be changed into 55° of average of louver angle.

The last rule is that it is assumed that the same group of the residents has similarity in their lifestyle. **Figure 14** shows an example of applying the louver control at the same angle after determining the average angle in the average louver direction of a similar group. The benefit of the third rule is that if you control according to a group of similar lifestyles, you are more likely to increase resident satisfaction. All of the abovementioned rules will be the same, but the third rule is more closely related to the concept of collective intellect.

Before

Resident	Residence Unit	Time	Façade Louver #	Louver Angle Before	Louver Angle After
D	4	12:00	4	5 →	45

(40 degree rotation)

❖ If the level of similarity in Behaviors =1.0

After

Resident	Residence Unit	Time	Façade Louver #	Louver Angle Before	Louver Angle After
A	1	12:00	1	30 →	45
E	5	12:00	5	5 →	45
J	9	12:00	9	5 →	45
L	11	12:00	11	15 →	45
M	12	12:00	12	10 →	45

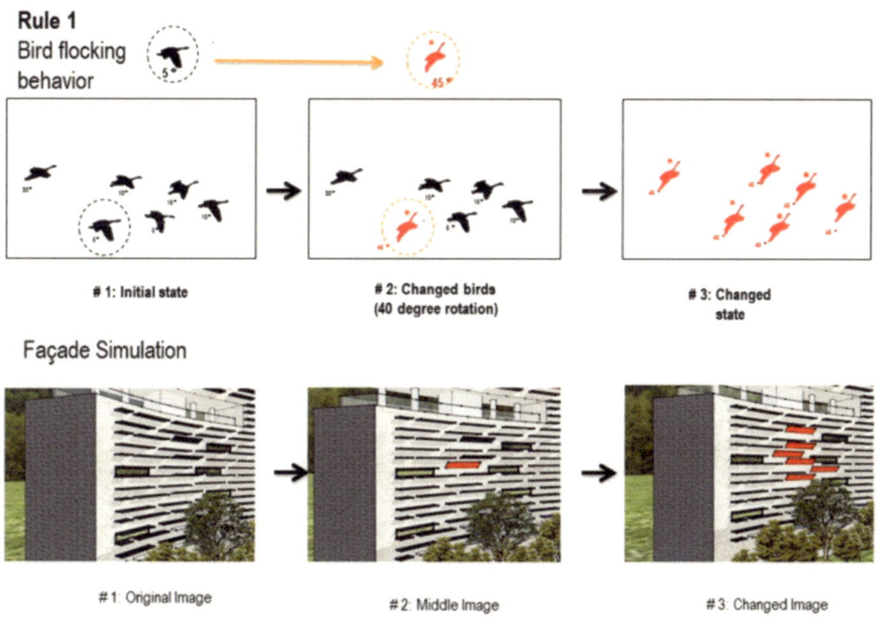

Figure 12. Façade simulation applied rule 1.

5.4. Discussion

In this study, we applied three biomimicry-inspired rules of behavior to a facade design. The method described here of applying the rules of bird behavior patterns to the case study building

Before

Resident	Residence Unit	Time	Façade Louver #	Louver Angle	
				Before	After
B	2	17:00	2	5 →	35

(30 degree rotation)

❖ If the level of similarity in Behaviors ≥ 0.8

After

Resident	Residence Unit	Time	Façade Louver #	Louver Angle	
				Before	After
C	3	17:00	3	30 →	60
D	4	17:00	4	20 →	50
F	6	17:00	6	10 →	40
G	7	17:00	7	5 →	35
K	11	17:00	11	15 →	45

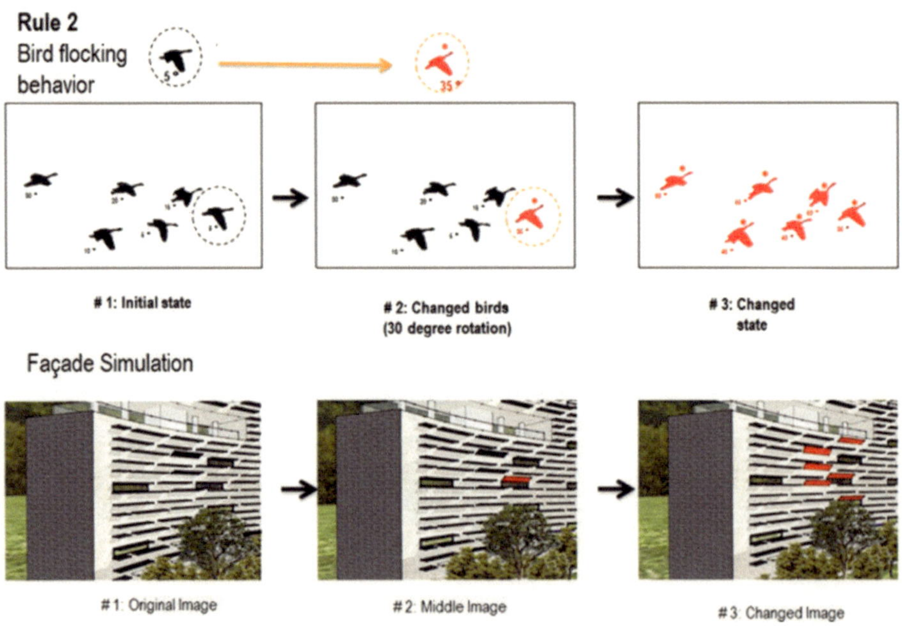

Figure 13. Façade simulation applied rule 2.

described here is surprisingly simple, indicating that it would be simple and straightforward to apply this method to the design of architectural facades. Significantly, the method also provides a starting point for one-to-one customized services based on lifestyle-driven rather than

http://dx.doi.org/10.5772/intechopen.72917

Before

Resident	Residence Unit	Time	Façade Louver #	Louver Angle	
				Before	After
A	1	18:00	1	20 →	80

❖ If the level of similarity in Behaviors =1.0

(Group 3)

User	Louver Angle	
	Before	After
A	20	80
D	10	35
H	5	45
J	30	60
(Group 3) Average		55

After

Resident	Residence Unit	Time	Façade Louver #	Louver Angle	
				Before	After
A	1	18:00	1	20 →	55
D	4	18:00	4	10 →	55
H	8	18:00	8	5 →	55
J	10	18:00	10	30 →	55

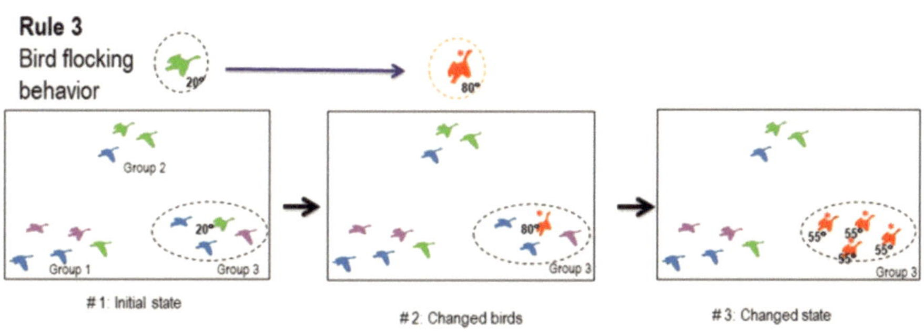

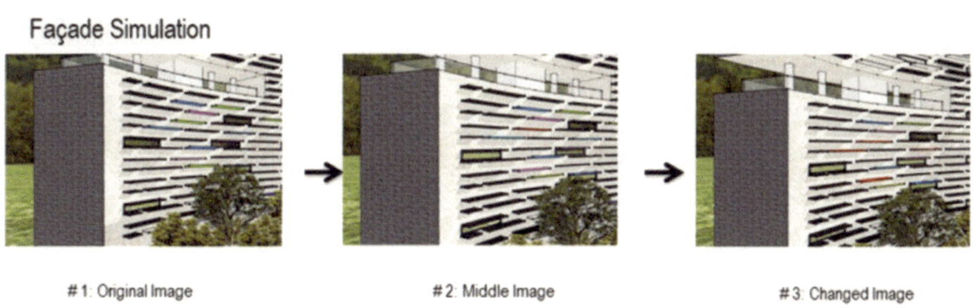

Figure 14. Façade simulation applied rule.

performance-driven controls. Performance-based controls can provide clear control baselines, but the problem is that the preference criteria for controls vary from resident to resident. One way to address this is through behavior-based control methods.

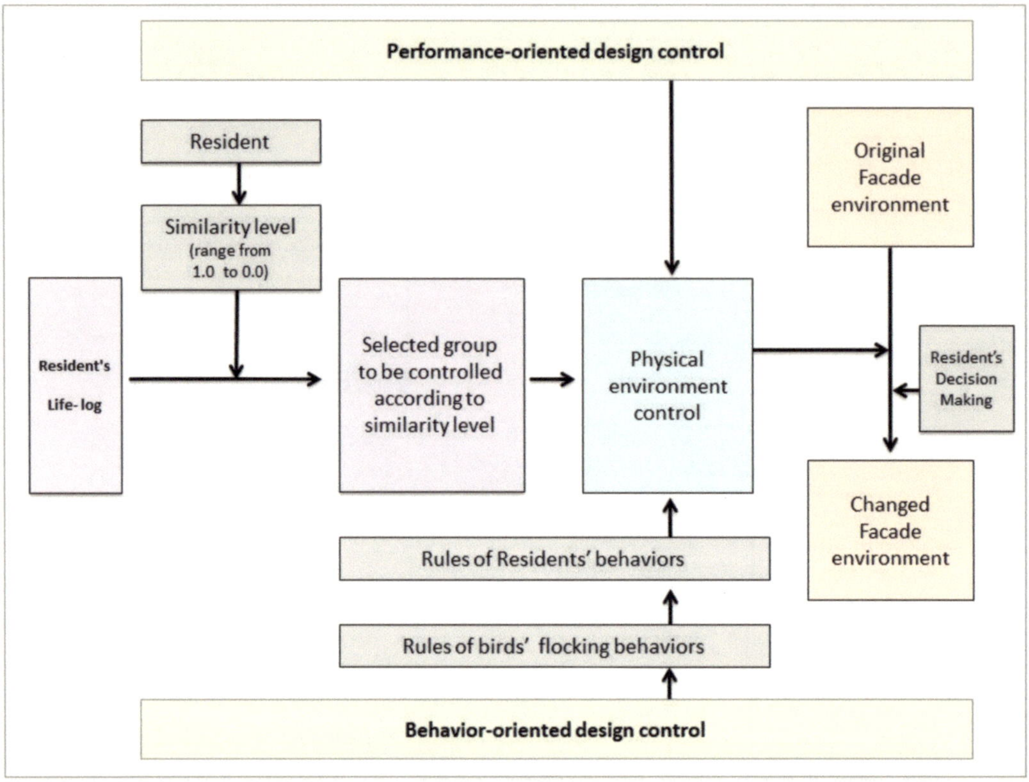

Figure 15. Hybrid control process of performance and behavior-based physical environment.

Above, we discussed the merits of biomimicry and also explained that biomimicry has a role in providing a source of design inspiration. The concept of biomimicry can take into account the form and function of any other natural organism. The present chapter focuses on the process of an adaptable façade design method for concept derivation, which still has practical limitations [9]. In the future research, more architectural sections and prototypes are needed to develop by adding more functional aspects. In other words, the development of intelligent façade louver controls requires a model that combines smart material and sensor technology rather than mechanical control. The ideal control process is a hybrid model that combines behavioral and performance bases, as shown in **Figure 15**.

6. Conclusion

6.1. Summary and contribution

This chapter focuses on adaptable architecture that responds to user behavior and the external environment, unlike previous studies on environmentally functional façades. In this regard, this chapter focuses on approaches to controlling façade functions based on user behavior and preference rather than a performance-based, functional control approach. The behavior-based method presented in this study provides an opportunity to increase the satisfaction of residents by providing each with individualized service. Of course, the behavior-based approach is not perfect. The ideal approach to façade control would be to integrate performance-based and behavior-based control methods more effectively.

The point of this chapter is not to mimic a bird's form but to apply principles of birds' behavior to an architectural façade. The contribution of this chapter is that it presents a façade louver control methodology based on an interpretation of birds' flight behavior from the perspective of facade louver control. In particular, this paper differs from the previous studies which has been focused on biological forms because it has viewed biomimicry in terms of biological processes and nature. Biomimetic design has great potential as a source of inspiration for innovative architectural design. A behavior-based approach, in particular, offers opportunities for users to increase their quality of life by meeting personalized needs.

6.2. Future research

In this study, a case study for the development of a façade design using biomimicry is presented. Although future research will propose an adaptable façade based on various façade types, this study limits itself to control of the façade louver angle. However, further research is needed to extend façade control to window opening and blind systems. Future research aimed at building a façade control system that considers the view of the interior from a user-centered rather than from an outside viewpoint is also needed.

Further research is also needed for further development of a hybrid façade that links performance and behavior. For instance, adaptable façades associated with ventilation, thermal insulation, and day lighting should be developed. Further studies on esthetic aspects of adaptable façades, including design algorithm patterns, composition, and design principles, should also be pursued. In addition, moving beyond planar façades, design methods for adaptable façades that fit curved forms must be developed. A study of adaptable façades that can be controlled by self-organism is also needed.

This chapter concludes that a good building should be able to respond flexibly to ever-changing environments. A bio-inspired adaptable façade is a solution with great potential for creating esthetically pleasing sustainable architecture with comfortable interior conditions.

Acknowledgements

This work was supported by the National Research Foundation of Korea (NRF) grant found by the Korean government(MOE) (NRF-2015-RlDlAlA09061276) and NRF Grant funded by Korean Government (NRF-2017-Fostering Core Leaders of the Future Basic Science Program/ Global Ph.D. Fellowship Program).

Author details

Hyunsoo Lee* and Nayeon Kim

*Address all correspondence to: hyunsl@yonsei.ac.kr

Department of Interior Architecture and Built Environment, Yonsei University, Seoul, South Korea

References

[1] Ball P. Follows your neighbour. In: Ball P, editor. Nature's Patterns. Oxford: Oxford University Press; 2009. pp. 124-159

[2] Beni G. From swarm intelligence to swarm robotics. In: SAB 2004 International Workshop on Swarm Robotics; July 17, 2005; Santa Monica. Berlin: Springer-Verlag; 2004. pp. 1-9

[3] Benyus JM. Biomimicry: Innovation Inspired by Nature. New York: Harper Collins Publishers; 2002

[4] Brownell B, Swackhamer M. Hypernatural: Architecture's New Relationship with Nature. New York: Princeton Architectural Press; 2015

[5] Caetano I, Leitão A. DrAFT: An algorithmic framework for facade design, generative design applications. Vol. 1. In: 34th CAADe; 2016; Oulu. pp. 465-474

[6] Capeluto G, Ochoa CE. Intelligent Envelopes for High-Performance Buildings: Design and Strategy. Switzerland: Springer; 2017. pp. 1-19

[7] Couzin ID, Krause J. Self-organization and collective behavior in vertebrates. Advances in the Study of Behavior. 2003;**32**:1-74

[8] Chen J, Huang S. Adaptive building facade optimization: An integrated green-BIM approach. In: 21st International Conference of the Association for Computer-Aided Architectural Design Research in Asia, CAADRIA; 2016; Hong Kong. pp. 259-268

[9] Fox M. Interactive Architecture: Adaptive World. New York: Princeton Architectural Press; 2016

[10] Fox M, Kemp M. Interactive Architecture. 1st ed. New York: Princeton Architectural press; 2009

[11] Gruber P. Biomimetics in Architecture: Architecture of Life and Buildings. Vienna: Ambra Verlag; 2010

[12] Harry S. Dynamic adaptive building envelopes: An innovative and state-of-the-art technology. Creative Space. 2016;**3**(2):167-183

[13] Helms M, Vattam SS, Goel AK. Biologically inspired design: Process and products. Design Studies. 2009;**30**:606-622

[14] Herzog T, Krippner R, Lang W. Facade Construct Manual. Basel: Boston, Birkhauser-Publishers for Architecture; 2004. pp. 36-47

[15] Kashani YA. Biomimetics and Architecture: An Exploration of Swarm Intelligence, Emergent Behaviour and Self-Organization. Saarbrucken: LAP Lambert Academic Publishing; 2012. pp. 57-70

[16] Kim E, Choi J. A case study on the environmental facade system using biomimicry. Proceedings of Conference of Architectural Institute of Korea. 2014;**34**(2):41-42

[17] Kolarevic B, Parlac V. Building Dynamics: Exploring Architecture of Change. London: Routledge; 2015

[18] Kotsopoulos SD, Casalegno F. Responsive architectures: Prototyping components and processes for the built environments of the late digital age, emerging experience in past, present and future of digital architecture. In: Proceedings of the 20th International Conference of the Association for Computer-Aided Architectural Design Research in Asia, CAADRIA; 2015; Hong Kong. pp. 335-344

[19] Lee H, Kim N. Biomimetic facade control inspired by bird flocking intelligence. In: Third International Conference of Biodigital Architecture & Genetics; 2017; Barcelona. pp. 38-49

[20] Lee H, Park S, Jung J. A study on developing a smart home service based on the behavior patterns of the elderly. Journal of the Architectural Institute of Korea Planning and Design. 2012;**28**(5):159-168

[21] Schmidt R, Austin S. Adaptable Architecture: Theory and Practice. London: Routledge; 2016

[22] Sjarifudin FU. Adaptive decorative building skin. In: 21st International Conference of the Association for Computer-Aided Architectural Design Research in Asia, CAADRIA; 2016; Hong Kong. pp. 425-434

[23] Pawlyn M. Biomimicry in Architecture. 2nd ed. Newcastle upon Tyne: Riba Publishing; 2016

[24] Pohl G, Nachtigall W. Biomimetics for Architecture & Design: Nature, Analogies, Technology. Cham: Springer; 2015

[25] Wu KY, Hao JH. Spark Wall: Control responsive environment by human behavior, emerging experience in past, present and future of digital architecture. In: Proceedings of the 20th International Conference of the Association for Computer-Aided Architectural Design Research in Asia, CAADRIA; Hong Kong. 2015

[26] Zeiny R. Biomimicry as a problem solving methodology in interior architecture. In: ASEAN Conference on Environment-Behaviour Studies; Bangkok. 2012. pp. 502-512

Chapter 7

Switchable and Reversible Superhydrophobic Surfaces: Part One

Sabri Taleb, Thierry Darmanin and Frédéric Guittard

Additional information is available at the end of the chapter

http://dx.doi.org/10.5772/intechopen.73022

Abstract

In this chapter, most of the methods used in the literature to prepare switchable and reversible superhydrophobic surfaces are described. Inspired by Nature, it is possible to induce the Cassie-Baxter–Wenzel transition using different external stimuli such as light, temperature, pH, ion exchange, voltage, magnetic field, mechanic stress, plasma, ultrasonication, solvent, gas or guest. Such properties are extremely important for various applications but especially for controllable oil/water separation membranes, oil-absorbing materials and water harvesting systems.

Keywords: superhydrophobic, reversible, switchable, bioinspiration, biomimetism

1. Introduction

Superhydrophobic surfaces are characterized by a water apparent contact angle (θ_w) above 150° and ultra-low water adhesion or hysteresis (H). The obtaining of superhydrophobic surfaces is crucial in a theoretical point of view and also for various applications such as in self-cleaning windows and textiles, antifingerprint or antireflective properties for optical instruments and mobile phones, liquid transportation, separation membrane, cell and antibacterial adhesion. In Nature, many plants and animals have superhydrophobic properties [1]. These surface properties are extremely important for example to survive against predators or in hostile or arid environments. One can cite the famous Lotus leaves with their self-cleaning properties and also other plants and animals able to slide on the water surface, to see in fogging environments, to walk on vertical substrates, to breath underwater or to swim very rapidly (**Figure 1**) [2–14].

For practical applications, it is often necessary to have "robust" superhydrophobic properties, which is possible combining appropriate surface structures and low surface energy materials.

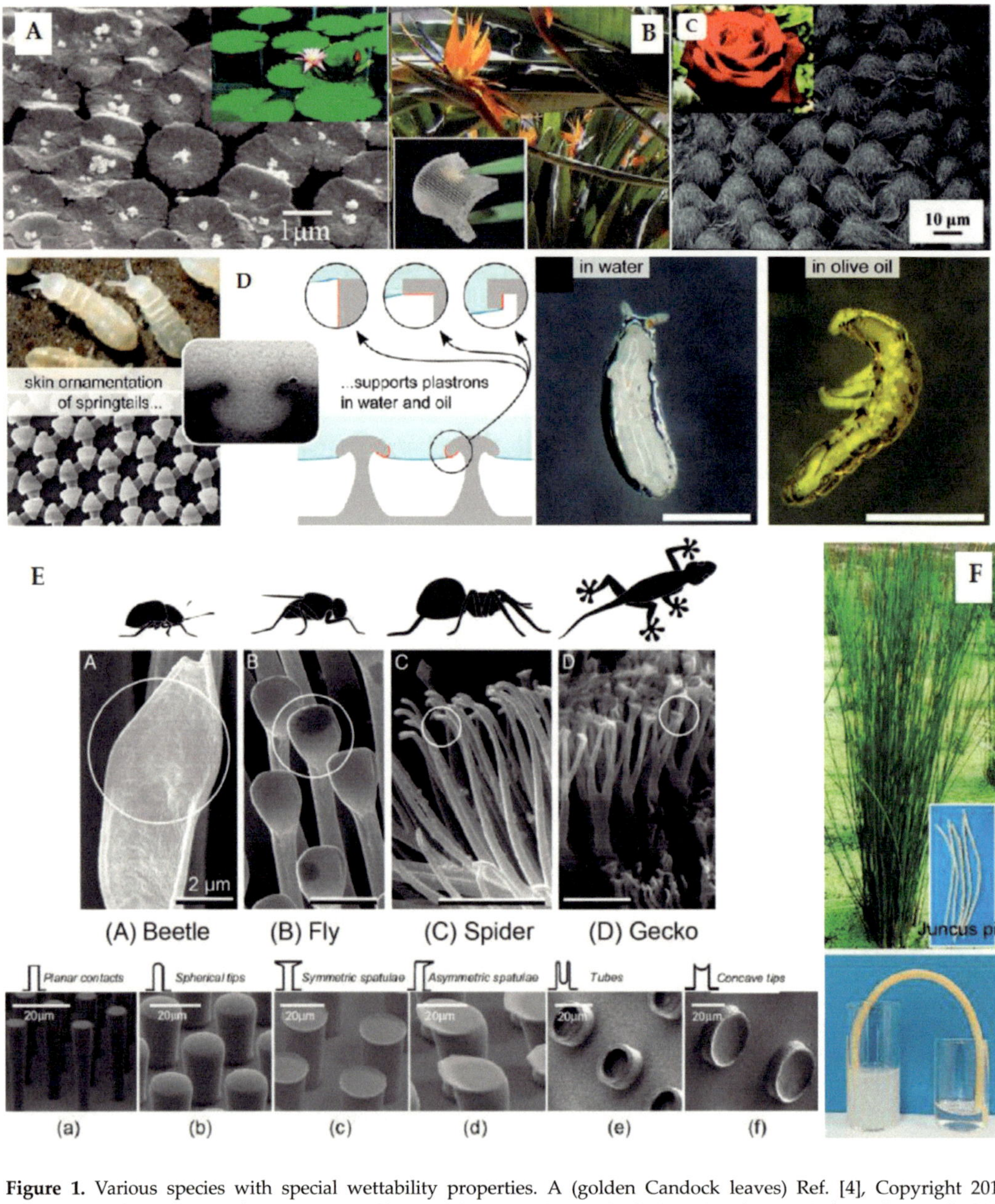

Figure 1. Various species with special wettability properties. A (golden Candock leaves) Ref. [4], Copyright 2011. Reprinted with permission from American Chemical Society, USA. B (*Strelitzia reginae* leaves) Ref. [5], Copyright 2012. Reprinted with permission from American Chemical Society, USA. C (rose petals) Ref. [9], Copyright 2008. Reprinted with permission from American Chemical Society, USA. D (springtails) Ref. [8], Copyright 2013. Reprinted with permission from American Chemical Society, USA. E (insect and animal foot) Ref. [13], Copyright 2009. Reprinted with permission from American Chemical Society, USA. F (Juncus pith) Ref. [14], Copyright 2017. Reprinted with permission from American Chemical Society, USA.

Indeed, robust superhydrophobic surfaces are obtained if the surface is able to stabilize the Cassie-Baxter state. Using an extern pressure, it is possible to induce the Cassie-Baxter–Wenzel transition but the transition is irreversible. Hence, in order to induce reversible Cassie-Baxter–Wenzel transition, extern stimuli are often used. In this chapter, most of the methods used in the literature to obtain switchable and reversible superhydrophobic surfaces are summarized. Indeed, different extern stimuli can be used such as the light, temperature, magnetic field, mechanical stress or ion exchange. Such materials are extremely used for applications in controllable oil/water separation membranes and water harvesting. One of the main applications is membranes with controllable wettability for oil/water separation. This application is extremely important to find solutions the spill of oil tankers. Another application is their use in car or building windows in order to see clearly even when it is raining. Water is also not wanted in building materials because it has a high thermal conductivity. Methods to remove quickly water are highly expected. Water harvesting is another important application and systems able to control water wettability are extremely promising especially in hot and arid environments.

2. Theoretical part

Both the surface energy (γ_{SV}) and the presence of surface roughness are key parameters to reach superhydrophobic properties. As reported by Young, the contact angles of a "smooth" substrate are governed by three surface tensions following the reaction: $\cos\theta^Y = (\gamma_{SV} - \gamma_{SL})/\gamma_{LV}$, where γ_{SV}, γ_{SL} and γ_{LV} are the surface tensions at the solid-vapor, solid-liquid and liquid-vapor interfaces, respectively [15]. However, the presence of surface roughness is fundamental to reach contact angles above 150°, as reported by Wenzel and Cassie-Baxter [16, 17] (**Figure 2**). These two equations take into account the effect of surface roughness, contrary to the Young equation but are also related to the Young equation. When the water droplet follows the Wenzel regime, it penetrates inside all the surface roughness leading to a full solid-liquid interface but amplified by the roughness parameter following the equation: $\cos\theta = r\cos\theta^Y$ (r is the roughness parameter) [16]. Hence, the adhesion of water droplet is important because the roughness parameter increases the solid-liquid interface. Moreover, it is possible to reach contact angle above 150° but only using intrinsically hydrophobic materials ($\theta^Y > 90°$). However, it is now admitted the possible to obtain superhydrophobic and even superoleophobic properties using intrinsically hydrophilic and oleophilic materials, respectively. This is possible only if air is present inside the surface roughness, as reported by Cassie-Baxter [17]. The Cassie-Baxter equation has to be applied when there is air trapped inside the surface roughness between the water droplet and the surface. The Cassie-Baxter equation is $\cos\theta = r_f f\cos\theta^Y + f - 1$ where r_f is the roughness ratio of the substrate wetted by the liquid, f the solid fraction and (1 − f) the air fraction. Moreover,

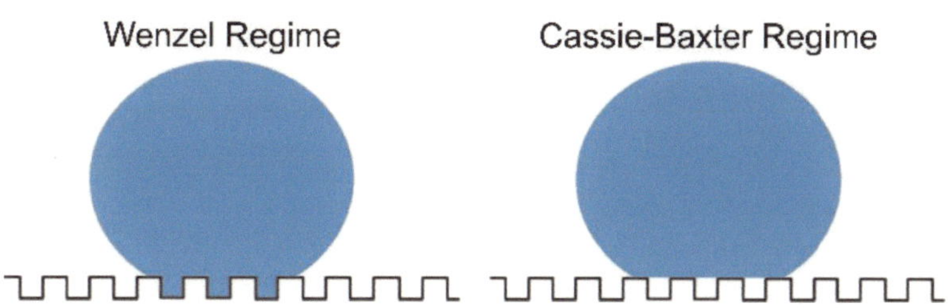

Figure 2. Schematic representation of a water droplet following the Wenzel and Cassie-Baxter equations.

with the Cassie-Baxter, it is possible to obtain superhydrophobic properties with ultra-low adhesion if the air fraction between the water droplet and the surface is extremely important.

The Wenzel and Cassie-Baxter are two extreme states, and it is possible to induce the Cassie-Baxter-to-Wenzel wetting transition by applying an extern pressure. Indeed, the Cassie-Baxter equation is a metastable state, and it is possible to switch from the Cassie-Baxter to the Wenzel state by supplying a sufficient energy. "Robust" superhydrophobic surfaces are surfaces that can repel water even if a high pressure is applied [18, 19]. This is the case of the lotus leaves, which remain superhydrophobic even during rainfalls. It was also shown that the presence of re-entrant surface structures often to increase the surface robustness [20–23]. However, the Cassie-Baxter-to-Wenzel wetting transition by applying an extern pressure is irreversible because the dewetting forces are too strong [24, 25]. In this review, by supplying other energies to the system, it will be shown how it is possible to obtain reversible Cassie-Baxter-to-Wenzel wetting transition with the possibility to obtain, for example, reversible superhydrophobic-to-superhydrophilic properties. Indeed, it is possible to obtain reversible superhydrophobic properties if this energy modifies the surface energy (γ_{SV}) and/or the surface roughness. Most of the extern stimuli used in the literature to obtain reversible superhydrophobic properties will be reviewed.

3. Reversible superhydrophobic surfaces

The surface energy and surface morphology are two main key parameters governing surface wettability. Extern stimuli are very interesting approaches to induce a change in surface energy and/or surface morphology and lead to a transition from hydrophobic/superhydrophobic to hydrophilic/superhydrophilic. The stimuli used in the literature will be described in order to induce reversible changes in surface wettability (**Figure 3**).

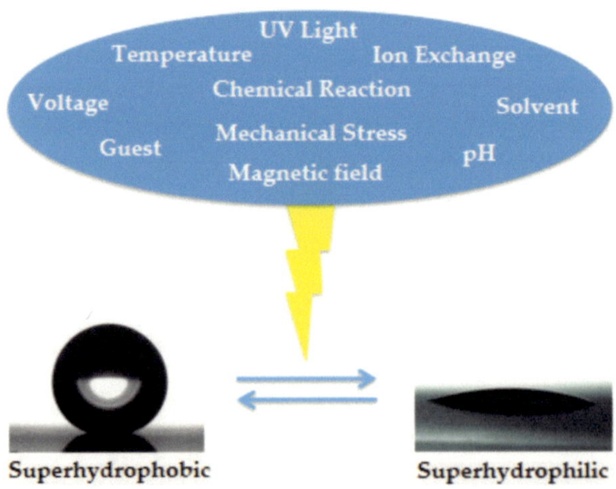

Figure 3. Schematic representation of reversible changes in the surface wettability using extern stimuli.

3.1. UV light

Light is one of the major extern stimuli used in the literature because of the easiness of utilization and high changes in surface wettability [26]. Various photosensitive inorganic oxides and organic polymers can undergo transitions from hydrophobic/superhydrophobic to hydrophilic/superhydrophilic after UV light irradiation and come back to the original state after storing in dark or exposing to visible light (VIS). This transition is often reversible during many cycles.

3.1.1. Inorganic materials

Among the photosensitive inorganic oxides, TiO_2 and ZnO are the most studied semiconductors. TiO_2 films are now largely used as steamtight and self-cleaning windows for their intrinsic photocatalytic properties and photo-induced hydrophilicity. Indeed, as shown in **Figure 4**, the presence of UV irradiation induces the formation of photoexcited electrons, which can reduce O_2 to generate superoxide radicals ($^{\bullet}O_2^-$) or hydroperoxyl radicals ($HO_2^{\bullet}$). These reactive oxygen species are able to convert organic pollutants into CO_2 and water and as a consequence clean the surface [27, 28].

In 1997, Watanabe et al. [29, 30] showed that the water contact angle (θ_w) of polycrystalline anatase TiO_2 was $72 \pm 1°$ and that their wettability properties could reversely change after UV light irradiation. Indeed, as shown in **Figure 4**, the surface of TiO_2 consists of oxygen bridges and UV irradiation creates oxygen vacancies converting Ti^{4+} into Ti^{3+}. These defects can then react with water forming hydrophilic group at the surface and as a consequence increase the surface hydrophilicity. Then, the wettability conversion was observed on both polycrystalline/monocrystalline anatase and rutile [31, 32]. Many works were dedicated to the modulation of the wettability of TiO_2 films [33, 34]. Among these works, low surface energy coatings were used to enhance the surface hydrophobicity. For example, the contact angle of colloidal crystal of TiO_2 films modified by fluoroalkylsilanes (FAS) was 100° [35]. Then, as observed in Nature, a huge attention was dedicated to the increase in surface roughness of TiO_2 films in order to obtain superhydrophobic properties ($\theta_w > 150°$ and low water adhesion). For example, based on Al_2O_3

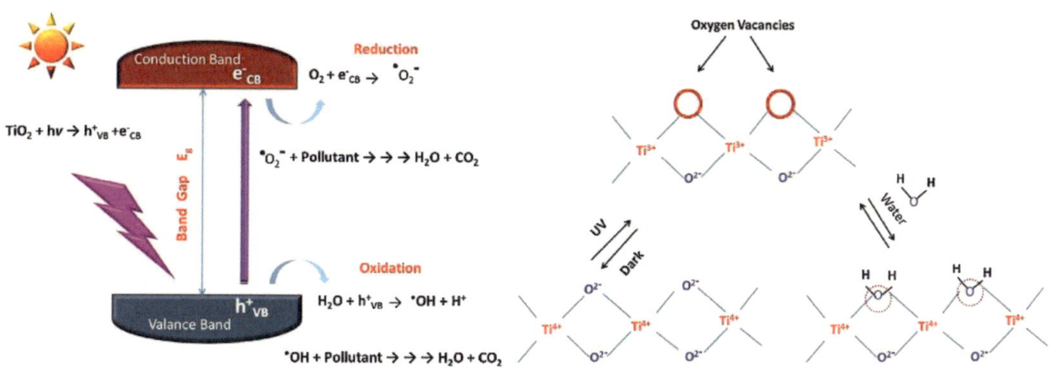

Figure 4. Left: Schematic representation of photocatalytic processes; right: schematic representation of photo-induced hydrophilicity, occurred during UV light irradiation of TiO_2.

colloids with flower-like morphology, rough colloidal TiO_2 films modified by fluoroalkylsilanes (FAS) was prepared in 2000 [36]. The combination of surface microstructures with low surface energy materials allowed reaching superhydrophobic properties with $\theta_w > 150°$. After exposure to UV light irradiation, the films became superhydrophilic with $\theta_w < 5°$.

Then, with the development of fabrication techniques, many processes were employed to obtain rough surface with various surface morphology [37–54]. TiO_2 nanorods with hierarchical dual-scale roughness were obtained using a hydrothermal process in the presence if TiO_3 and NaCl. The surfaces displayed superhydrophobic properties with $\theta_w = 154 \pm 1.3°$ without using low surface energy materials and superhydrophilic properties with $\theta_w \approx 0°$ after UV light irradiation. Moreover, after dark storage, the surface properties could reversely change from superhydrophobic to superhydrophilic during different cycles [37].

Vertically aligned TiO_2 nanotubes were also reported by anodization of Ti substrates in the presence of F^- [38–40]. The tube diameter and length were 175 nm and 3.3 μm, while the density of TiO_2 the nanotubes was 2.3×10^7 tubes mm^{-2}. After modification with a fluoroalkylsilane, the substrates displayed superhydrophobic properties with low water adhesion before UV irradiation and parahydrophobic with high water adhesion after UV irradiation. Moreover, the substrates could reversely switch from non-sticky to sticky by UV irradiation and heat annealing. Other authors also report the possible switching from highly hydrophobic and superhydrophilic using *N*-doped TiO_2 nanotubes but without low surface energy materials (**Figure 5**) [39]. Superhydrophobic TiO_2 surfaces with nanostrawberry-like morphology were also reported using a seeding growth process [41].

Now, TiO_2-based superhydrophobic surfaces with reversibility are largely used for the conception of smart surfaces and other functional materials. However, some rough morphologies lead to a severe dispersion of the light if their roughness is higher than the wavelength of the light and as a consequence to a loss in transparency. Hence, a promising strategy is the use of surfaces with low surface roughness [42]. In order to obtain an easy and reproducible method, Fujishima et al.

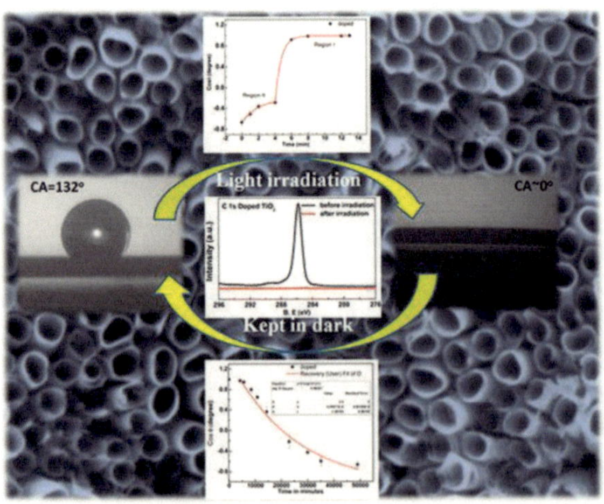

Figure 5. TiO_2 nanotubes with reversible wetting properties upon UV light irradiation and dark storage. Ref. [39], copyright 2013. Reprinted with permission from American Chemical Society, USA.

used a CF_4 plasma etching to reach microstructured TiO_2-based superhydrophobic properties [43, 44] after coating with octadodecylphosphonic acid (ODP). After an etching time of 30s, surfaces with $\theta_w > 165°$ were obtained with reversible conversion by UV irradiation. Ti substrates with switchable and reversible wettability from underwater superoleophobic to superoleophilic were also obtained by femtolaser laser treatment. The substrates are excellent candidates for separating oil/water mixtures [45]. TiO_2 nanoparticles were also deposited on microstructured surfaces in order to enhance the surface properties [45–54]. For example, Franssila et al. used substrates with microscale overhang pillars before depositing TiO_2 nanoparticles by atomic layer deposition [46, 47]. Depending on the UV irradiation time, the surfaces could switch from superhydrophobic to parahydrophobic (1 min), hydrophilic (5 min) or superhydrophilic (10 min). TiO_2 nanoparticles were also deposited on pre-patterned substrates such as paper, membranes or sponges in order to induce different special wettabilities [51–54].

ZnO is another extremely important photosensitive semiconductor for its intrinsic optical, electronic and acoustic properties, reacting similarly to TiO_2 [55, 56]. Here, also many works were dedicated to induce ZnO structures with high roughness [57–79]. Jiang et al. reported the obtaining of ZnO nanorod arrays using hydrothermal processes (**Figure 6**). Their diameter and length were 50–150 nm and 1.2 μm, respectively. The surfaces displayed switchable and reversible properties from superhydrophobic ($\theta_w = 161.2°$) to superhydrophilic by alternating UV light irradiation and dark storage [57]. These kinds of materials could also be used as memristors controllable with the illumination direction [60].

Another application is the preparation of controllable membranes for oil/water separation with specific wetting properties. For example, Jiang et al. developed switchable and reversible superhydrophobic-superhydrophilic and underwater superoleophobic properties by growth of ZnO nanorods on stainless steel meshes (**Figure 7**). More precisely, the meshes were both superhydrophobic and underwater superoleophilic but became both superhydrophilic and underwater superoleophobic after UV light irradiation [61].

ZnO nanorods were also reported using other processes, including chemical vapor deposition (CVD) [62], spray [63, 64] or electrodeposition [65, 66]. Otherwise, ZnO nanostructures of various shapes, including nanosheets, nanowires or nanoflowers, can be easily produced [67–77]. For example, nanoflower structures were obtained just by adding NH_3 during the hydrothermal process in order to form $Zn(NH_3)_4^{2+}$ complexes before the formation of ZnO structures [76]. ZnO nanowires were also reported by annealing Zn films at 500°C [70]. Otherwise, the growth of ZnO can also be induced on pre-structured surfaces. For example, a smooth ZnO film was added to Si nanospikes to reach reversible wettability and photocatalytic behavior [78, 79].

Various other oxides, including WO_3, V_2O_5, SnO_2, CuO, Fe_2O_3, In_2O_3, SiC and GaN, were used to reversibly change the surface wettability from superhydrophobic to superhydrophilic by alternating UV light irradiation and dark storage or heat treatment [80–92]. For example, Wang et al. showed that the protein adsorption and cell adhesion on GaN nanowires can be modulated by UV irradiation because the surface wettability changes from superhydrophobic to superhydrophilic. It was also sometimes necessary to add a hydrophobic molecule to enhance the surface hydrophobicity and the UV treatment is often able to remove this molecule [93–97]. For example, Bi_2O_3 hyperbranched dendritic structures were superhydrophobic but only after immersion in stearic acid solution [96]. Then, the UV irradiation was able to remove stearic acid

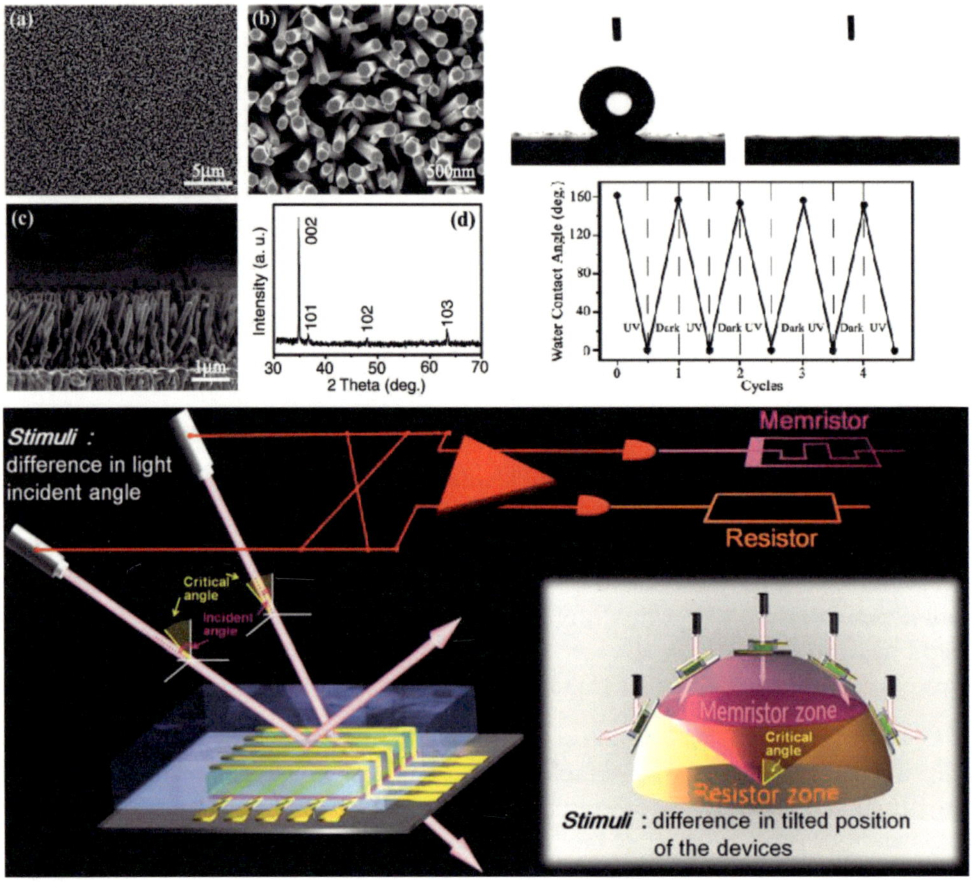

Figure 6. ZnO nanorod arrays with reversible wetting properties upon UV light irradiation and dark storage. The panels a-d represent FE-SEM top-images at low and high magnifications, cross-sectional view and XRD pattern of the ZnO nanorod films. The materials were used as controllable memristors. Ref. [57, 96], Copyright 2004. Reprinted with permission from American Chemical Society, USA [60].

and the surface became superhydrophilic. However, to obtain superhydrophobic properties again, it was necessary to add stearic acid again.

Similarly, carbon-based materials, including carbon nanotubes and graphene films, were also found to change from superhydrophobic to superhydrophilic by UV light irradiation and dark storage [98–101]. Here, the authors proposed that UV irradiation allows to change the absorbed O_2 molecules into hydrophilic groups such as hydroxyl ones [98]. Moreover, various inorganic oxides (such ZnO, p-Si, Al_2O_3, $SrTiO_3$, Sn, ZnS, CuO, Ag_2O and Cr_2O_3) were found to be also sensitive to X-ray with reversible wettability [102].

3.1.2. Nanocomposites

In order to enhance the stability of the light-sensitive materials, nanocomposites are often performed [103–114]. For example, superhydrophobic TiO_2/polystyrene (PS) nanocomposites were prepared in the literature. The material wettability could be reversely switch from

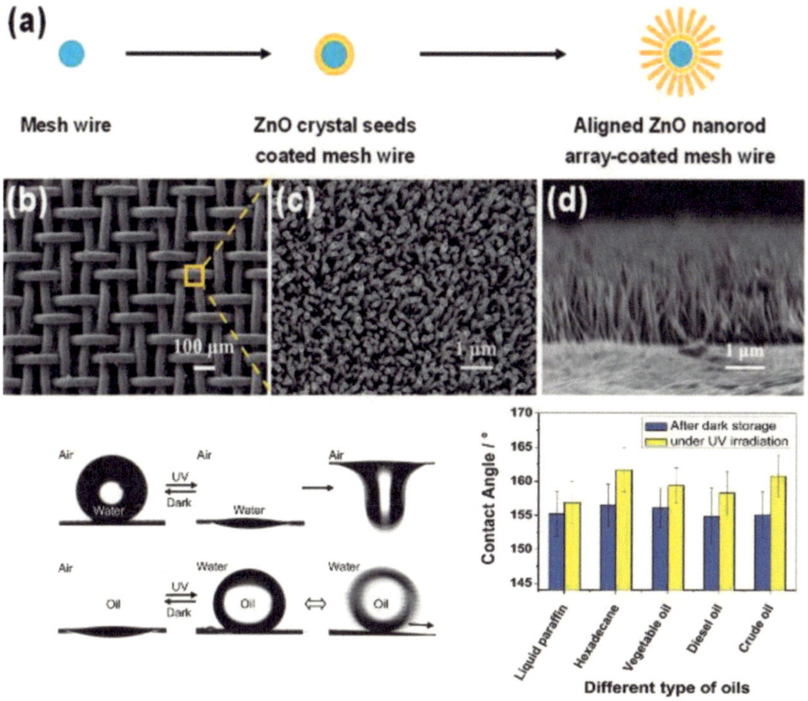

Figure 7. ZnO nanorod arrays grown on stainless steel meshes (Panel A). The Panels b-d represent SEM top view, local enlarged view and side view of the aligned ZnO nanorod array-coated stainless steel mesh film. The resulting meshes could switch from superhydrophobic and underwater superoleophilic to superhydrophilic and underwater superoleophobic upon UV light irradiation. Ref. [61], Copyright 2012. Reprinted with permission from Royal Society of Chemistry, United Kingdom.

superhydrophobic to superhydrophilic by alternating UV light illumination and heat treatment [103, 104]. Using Ag-TiO_2/poly(methyl methacrylate) (PMMA) nanocomposites, it was also possible to switch from superhydrophobic (low adhesion) to parahydrophobic (high adhesion) after UV irradiation [105]. Moreover, the materials displayed anticorrosive properties. ZnO/polyurethane (PU) nanocomposites were also sprayed on stainless steel meshes [110]. The resulting meshes displayed superhydrophobic and superhydrophilic/underwater superoleophobic properties by alternating UV treatment and heat treatment. These meshes could be used to separate oil/water mixtures. Chen et al. also used $TiO_2 - SiO_2$/polydimethylsiloxane (PDMS) to coat polyester-cotton fabrics [111]. The resulting fabrics were wash-resistant, resistant to strong acids and could be used to separate oil/water mixtures. Moreover, the photocatalytic properties of TiO_2 were also useful to treat dye waste water. Fluorinated compounds or polymers can also be used in order to enhance the superhydrophobic properties [112–114]. For example, TiO_2/poly(vinylidene fluoride) (PVDF) displayed both extremely high $\theta_w = 160.1°$ and low sliding angle (5.5°), and anticorrosive properties [112].

3.1.3. Photochromic organic groups

Organic chemicals containing photochromic functional groups such as azobenzenes [115], diarylethenes, spiropyrans [116], bipyridyl ethylenes [117], stilbenes [118] or pyrimidines [119] can follow a reversible transition by UV/vis light, which can lead to differences of wettability.

Among them, azobenzene group and its derivatives are extremely promising as photosensitive materials and were highly studied in the literature [120–135]. The azobenzene group is able to reversely switch from the *trans* to the *cis* isomer by UV light and visible light irradiation, as shown in **Figure 8** [121]. After grafting azobenzene on a polymer, Jiang et al. reported that the *trans* isomer is more hydrophobic because it has a smaller dipole moment and a low surface energy, in comparison to the *cis* isomer. Indeed, the benzene substituent is more present at the extreme surface in the *trans* isomer. However, the changes in θ_w on smooth substrates are lower than 10° after UV irradiation [122].

In 2005, Jiang et al. prepared a rough micro-patterned silicon substrate by photolithography and deposited on it a monolayer of azobenzene [121]. They showed that the difference in θ_w between the *trans* and *cis* isomer is highly depending on the spacing between the pillars (**Figure 9**). The highest θ_w difference was obtained for a spacing of 40 μm, for which a change from 152.6 to 78.3° was observed after UV light irradiation. Hence, the maximal difference observed was 66.3°.

In order to enhance the surface properties, hydrophobic substituents such as CF_3 were grafted on the benzene ring of azobenzene groups [123]. When azobenzene is in the *trans* form, the CF_3 groups are at the extreme surface and the surface is expected to be more hydrophobic than without CF_3 groups. Combining fluorinated azobenzene with high roughness, Cho et al. were

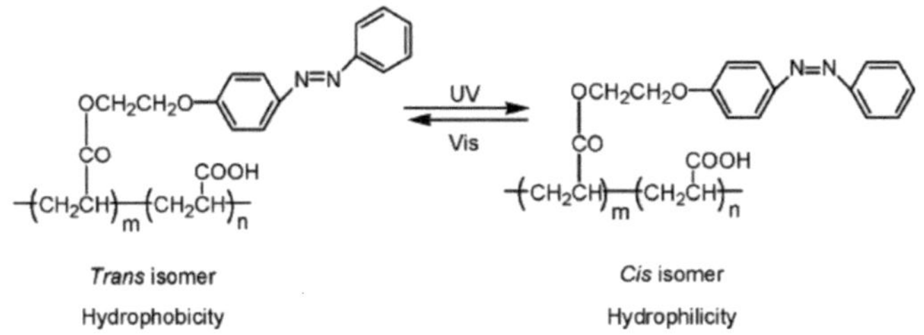

Figure 8. Reversible change in the *cis-trans* configuration of azobenzene group upon UV light and visible light irradiation. Ref. [121], Copyright 2005. Reprinted with permission from Royal Society of Chemistry, United Kingdom.

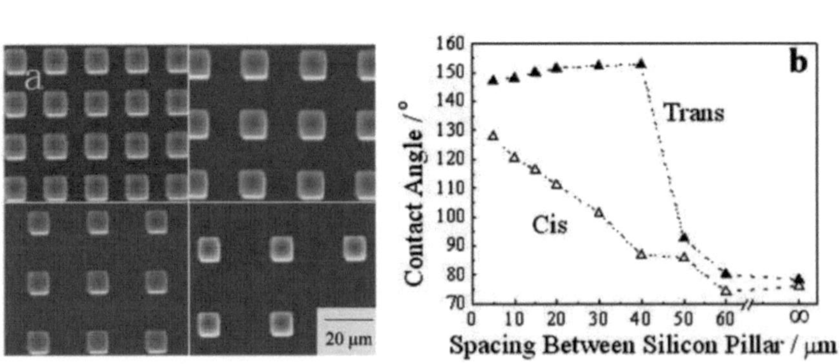

Figure 9. Variation of the water contact angle (Panel B) of a monolayer of azobenzene deposited on a micro-patterned silicon substrate as a function of the pillar spacing (Panel A). Ref. [121], Copyright 2005. Reprinted with permission from Royal Society of Chemistry, United Kingdom.

the first to show the possibility reversibly switch from superhydrophobic to superhydrophilic during the *trans/cis* transition [124, 125]. Using a layer-by-layer strategy alternating poly (allylamine hydrochloride) (PAH) and SiO_2 nanoparticles to obtain rough surfaces, the azobenzene substituents were grafted during the last step. Even if the UV irradiation induced a small θ_w difference (5°) for the smooth substrate, the increase in roughness induces a huge θ_w difference up to 147° for nine deposition cycles. Similar results were obtained using core-shell $Fe_3O_4@SiO_2$ nanoparticles [126]. The surface hydrophobicity could be easily controlled with the UV or visible light illumination time (**Figure 10**). These materials could also be used to selectively induce water permeation inside membranes.

Other works showed the possibility to modify cotton and paper substrates with these kinds of photosensitive polymers [127–129]. Using polyhedral oligomeric silsesquioxane (POSS) and fluorinated azobenzene, Gao et al. reported the possibility to obtain cotton fabrics with switchable from superhydrophobic/superoleophobic to highly hydrophobic/oleophobic [128, 129]. Indeed, many works were dedicated to the switching from superhydrophobic (low adhesion) to parahydrophobic (high adhesion) after UV irradiation. In order to achieve these properties, many strategies were employed in the literature [130–135]. For example, Xu et al. used an organotellurium-mediated controlled radical polymerization (TERP) in order to achieve polymers

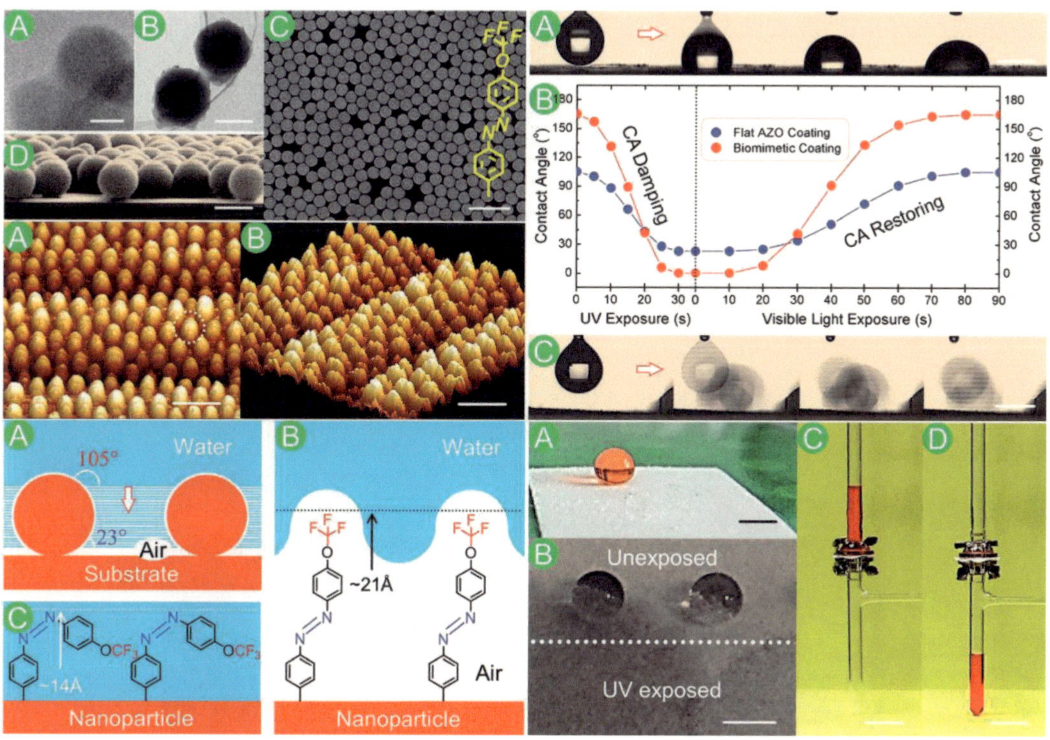

Figure 10. Preparation of light-induced water permeation membranes by grafting azobenzene with CF_3 groups on $Fe_3O_4@SiO_2$ nanoparticles. Ref. [126], Copyright 2014. Reprinted with permission from Royal Society of Chemistry, United Kingdom.

with micro/nanostructures [130–132]. Hu et al. used SiO_2 nanoparticles and polydopamine in order to graft the azobenzene moieties on SiO_2 nanoparticles [131]. By contrast, other groups deposited azobenzene-based materials on pre-structured surfaces [133–135]. For example, Rühe et al. deposited the azobenzene moieties on Si nanograss obtained by etching Si substrates with C_4F_8, SF_6 and O_2. The surfaces could switch from low adhesion to completely sticky after UV irradiation [133]. Yu et al. used micro and nanostructures substrates obtained by photolithography and etching before depositing the azobenzene moieties [134]. The authors measured an adhesion force of 60.6 ± 12.3 μN and 80.8 ± 4.9 μN before and after UV illumination, respectively. Liu et al. used anodized aluminum substrates with a "building blocks" morphology. After coating with a PDMS polymer grafted with azobenzene moieties, the substrates displayed switchable wettability from superhydrophobic (low adhesion: 6.2 μN for the *trans* isomer) to parahydrophobic (high adhesion: 44.8 μN for the *cis* isomer) properties after UV irradiation [135].

Diarylethene derivatives were found to be another excellent choice for light-sensitive switchable wettability (**Figure 11**). In this case, the light induces a change in the chemical structure from open-ring isomer to closed ring isomer. Uchida et al. reported the unique behavior of this molecule. Upon UV light irradiation, the film became superhydrophobic with $\theta_w = 163°$ due to the formation of microfibrils of diameter around 1 μm [136, 137]. Upon visible light irradiation, the surface again became flat with $\theta_w = 120°$. The chemical structure of the diarylethene can also be changed in order to modify the microcrystalline structures. For example, the surface morphology could be modified by sulfonation of the thiophene rings [138].

Different substituents were also introduced to change the material crystallinity [139–141]. The authors demonstrated that in order to obtain superhydrophobic properties with $\theta_w > 170°$, it is preferable to form densely submicrometer sized needle-shaped crystals [139]. For that, it is important that the eutectic temperature of the two isomers of the diarylethene is above that the temperature of formation. Otherwise, large crystals are formed (**Figure 12**).

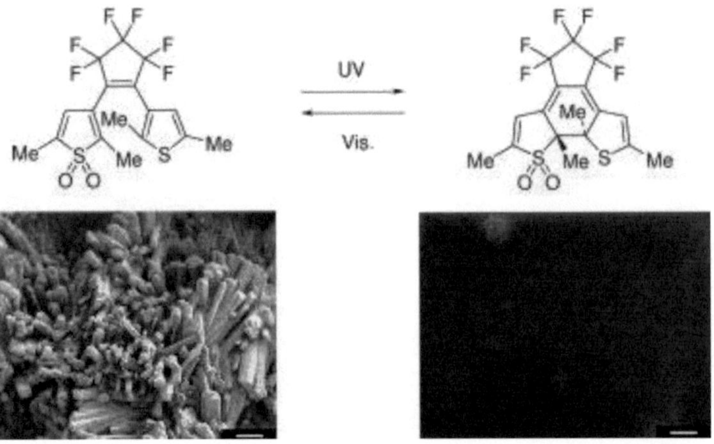

Figure 11. Reversible change of diarylethene from smooth open-ring isomer to microfibers of closed ring isomer upon UV light irradiation. Ref. [138], Copyright 2011. Reprinted with permission from American Chemical Society, USA.

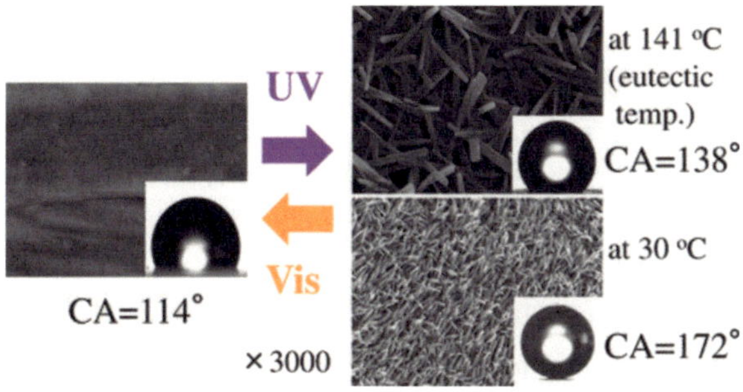

Figure 12. Influence of the eutectic temperature of the diarylethene-type molecule of the parameters of the formed crystals. Ref. [139], Copyright 2012. Reprinted with permission from American Chemical Society, USA.

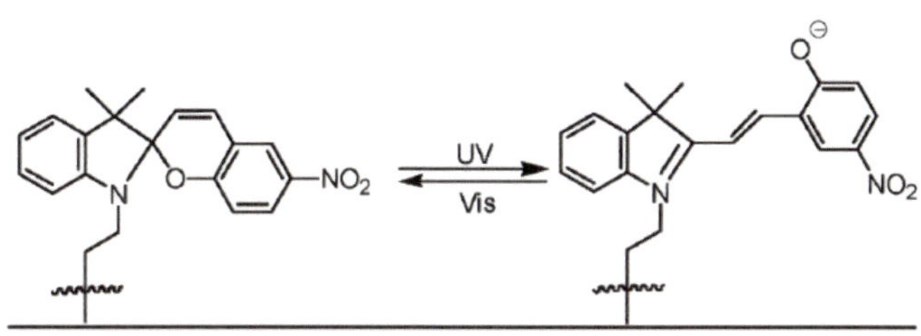

Figure 13. Reversible change in the form of spiropyran upon UV light and visible light irradiation. Ref. [142], Copyright 2002. Reprinted with permission from American Chemical Society, USA.

Spiropyran is another kind of photochromic organic moiety with wetting properties sensitive to light. Its closed form is apolar and hydrophobic, whereas its open form is polar and hydrophilic (**Figure 13**). These two forms can be reversely switched by UV and visible light irradiation [142–144].

In order to obtain superhydrophobic, spiropyran-based molecules can be deposited on rough surface [145–148]. For example, the deposition on Si nanograss gave rise to superhydrophobic properties. Moreover, the authors observed a change from superhydrophobic (low adhesion) to parahydrophobic (high adhesion) properties upon UV light irradiation [145]. Smirnov et al. also reported the possible control of water into a nanoporous aluminum membrane containing a spiropyran moiety using light [147]. Here, the photosensitive membrane acts as a burst valve, allowing the transport of water and ions across the membrane. Lu et al. also reported the formation of melamine-formaldehyde sponge with spiropyran moiety for oil recovery. The sponge was able to control oil absorption and desorption under light illumination [148].

Coumarin was also used in the literature to change the surface wettability. Here, the UV light induces the dimerization of coumarin as shown in **Figure 14**. Hampp et al. deposited a self-assembled monolayer (SAM) with coumarin moieties [149]. They observed a change of θ_w from 70 to 55°. Xu et al. grafted coumarin on SiO_2 nanoparticles [150]. The authors observed in a change of the surface morphology from random nanoparticle aggregates to rings accompanied with a change of θ_w from 102 to 163°.

3.2. Temperature

The reversibility of surface wettability by thermal treatment has given rise to a huge interest during the last years [151, 152]. Poly(*N*-isopropylacrylamide) (PNIPAAm) has been extensively used as an example polymer with thermal response, which has a low critical solution temperature (LCST) of around 32–33°C [151]. On smooth substrate, the θ_w of modified PNNIPAAm can changed from hydrophilic to hydrophobic when the temperature is over LCST, resulting from competition between intra- and intermolecular interactions, as shown in **Figure 15**.

By grafting the polymer on rough silicon surface obtained by etching, the surface wettability could be changed from superhydrophilic to superhydrophobic with θ_w = 149.3° when the

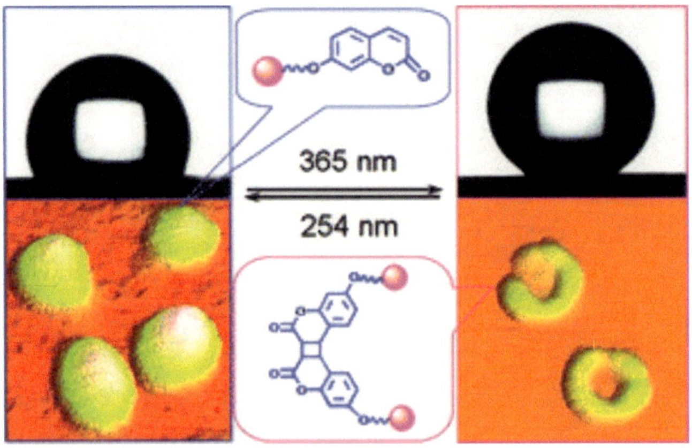

Figure 14. Reversible change of coumarin from aggregates of monomers to rings of dimers upon UV light and visible light irradiation. Ref. [150], Copyright 2012. Reprinted with permission from Royal Society of Chemistry, United Kingdom.

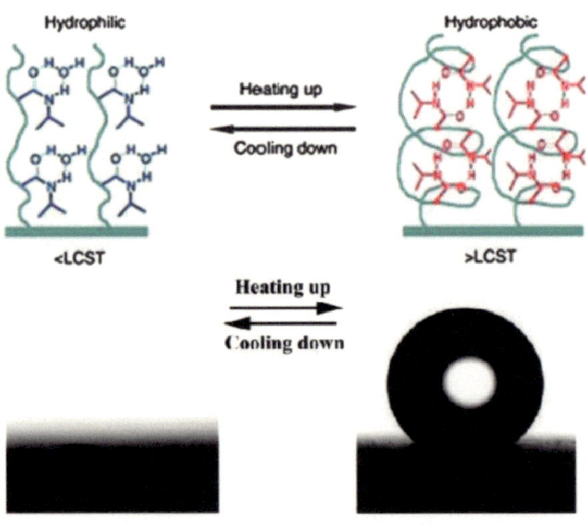

Figure 15. Influence of heating on the intra- and intermolecular interactions in PNNIPAAm and the resulting surface hydrophobicity [151].

temperature changed from 25 to 40°C. Other works also reported this possibility using different strategies [153–156].

PNIPAAm/PS and PNIPAAm/poly(*L*-lactide) (PLLA) nanocomposites were also produced by electrospinning [157, 158]. Depending on the concentration of the constituents, the surface morphology could be changed from beads to long nanofibers. At high concentration of PNIPAAm, the surface could change from superhydrophilic to superhydrophobic when the temperature changed from 20 to 50°C. It was also shown that the response time to switch is depending on the size of the fibers [159]. When the diameter of the fiber was small (around 380–1500 nm), the response time was 4–5 s [160]. Other nanocomposites were also reported with this technique. PNIPAAm/PS blends were used to obtain densely packed nanocupules of 284 nm diameter and 31 nm wall thickness using an anodized aluminum oxide (AAO) template (**Figure 16**) [161]. Here, the surface could switch by changing the temperature from parahydrophobic (high adhesion) to superhydrophobic (low adhesion) with a difference in adhesion force of around 20 μN.

PNIPAAm was also polymerized on an elastic polyurethane (PU) microfibrous membrane by free radical polymerization [162]. The membrane could be used for controllable oil/water separation. At 25°C, the membrane was underwater superoleophobic, while at 45°C the membrane was underwater superoleophilic (**Figure 17**).

Xin et al. reported the preparation of PNIPAAm-cotton fabrics able to collect different amount of water from fog [163]. At room temperature, the cotton showed a water uptake of 340%, while at 40°C the uptake was only 24%. Such materials are extremely interesting for water harvesting systems. Microfluidic thermosensitive valves were also prepared [164, 165]. After coating with PNIPAAm, the valve was hydrophilic at room temperature and allowed the flow (opening status), while at 70°C, the valve was superhydrophobic and stopped the water flow

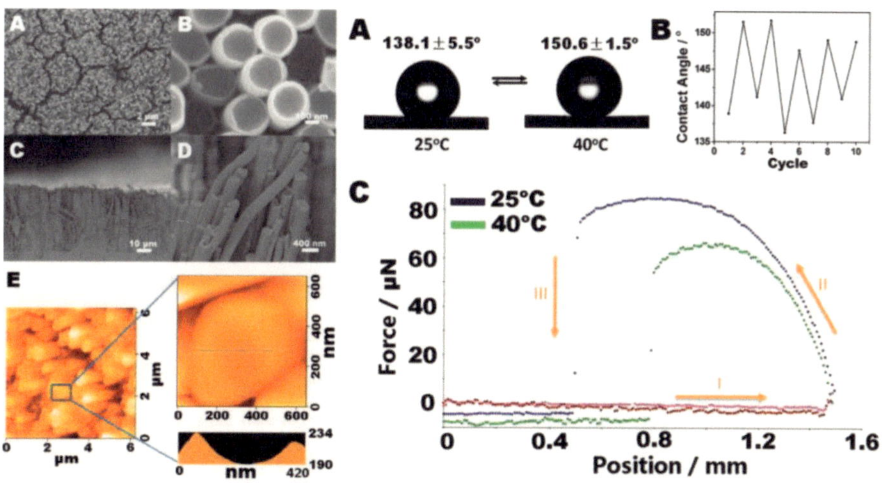

Figure 16. Densely packed PNIPAAm/PS blends nanocupules with reversible change from superhydrophobic (low adhesion) to parahydrophobic (high adhesion) by heating and cooling. Ref. [161], Copyright 2014. Reprinted with permission from Royal Society of Chemistry, United Kingdom.

(closing status). Using a similar idea, an "ON-OFF" switchable enzymatic biofuel cell was reported [166]. Here, gold nanoparticles protected glucose oxidase and laccase were entrapped into PNIPAAm chains. At room temperature, the fuels and the mediator could access to the catalytic centers of enzymes ("ON" state), while at 50°C the process of reactant transmission was blocked ("OFF" state).

Poly(ε-caprolactone) (PCL) was also tested as a thermosensitive polymer with a transition from crystalline phase to amorphous phase (**Figure 18**) [167]. Jiang et al. showed that PCL_{10000} is an ideal material. For a smooth surface, θ_w of PCL_{10000} was 88.1°C at room temperature because the polymer chains are frozen by crystallization. However, at 60°C, θ_w was 60.8°C because water can induce the reorientation of the hydrophobic/hydrophilic groups. Moreover, by depositing this polymer rough substrate composed of arrays of square pillars (10 μm × 10 μm in width, 30 μm in height), a change from superhydrophobic to superhydrophilic was observed after heat treatment. The highest properties were obtained groove spacing of 40 μm.

SiO_2 and carbon nanotube/PCL nanocomposites were also used in the literature [168, 169]. For example, using carbon nanotubes, it was reported the possibility to switch from hydrophobic to hydrophilic or from superhydrophobic (low water adhesion) to parahydrophobic (high water adhesion), dependent on PCL concentration.

Liquid crystalline polymers also showed thermosensitivity when the temperature induces a reversible change from liquid crystalline to isotrope. After grafting liquid crystalline segments (butyl-oxy biphenylcarbonitrile) on a smooth PDMS elastomer, the authors observed a change of θ_w from 92.4 to 89.3° due to a change of the polymer from smectic A to isotrope [170]. The same polymer was also used to cover rough substrates composed of arrays of square pillars (10 μm × 10 μm in width,

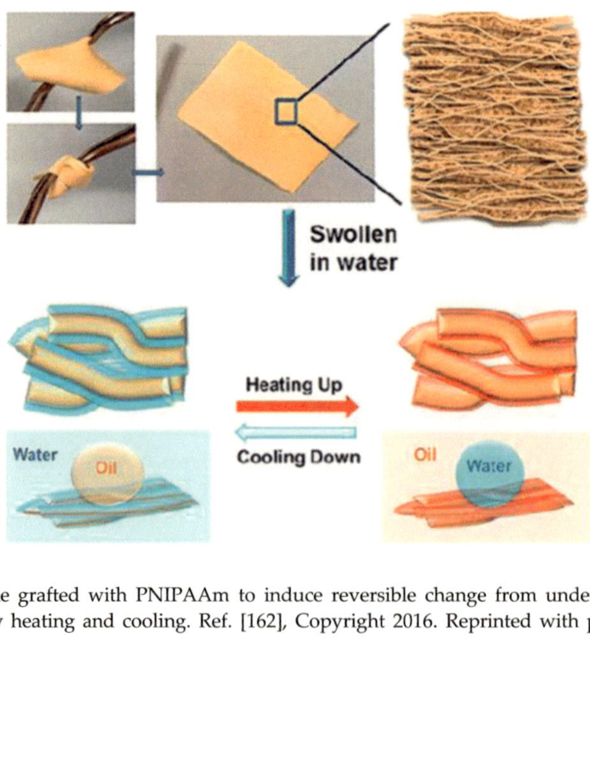

Figure 17. PU membrane grafted with PNIPAAm to induce reversible change from underwater superoleophobic to underwater oleophilic by heating and cooling. Ref. [162], Copyright 2016. Reprinted with permission from American Chemical Society, USA.

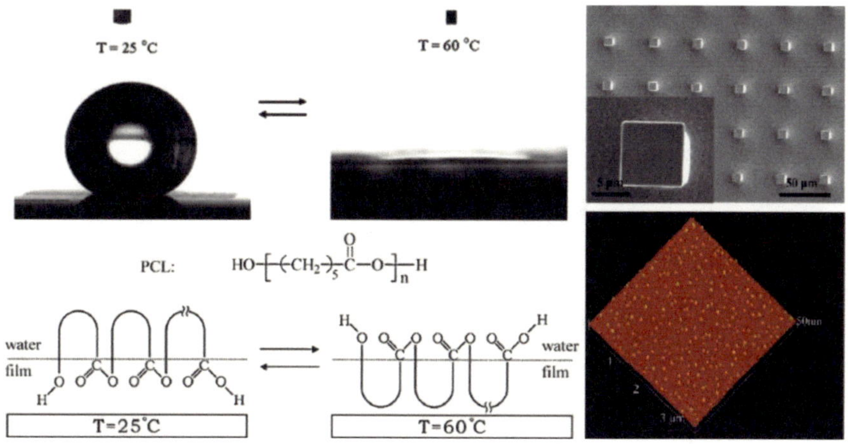

Figure 18. Influence of heating on the phase transition from crystalline to amorphous of PCL_{10000} and the resulting surface hydrophobicity. Ref. [167], Copyright 2008. Reprinted with permission from Royal Society of Chemistry, United Kingdom.

30 μm in height). A huge influence of the groove spacing was observed. Interestingly, a change from superhydrophobic (low water adhesion) to parahydrophobic (high water adhesion) was observed for a groove spacing of 15 μm. Liquid crystalline elastomers were also prepared using a side-on liquid crystalline monomer 4″-acryloyloxybutyl 2,5-di(4′-butyloxybenzoyloxy)benzoate [171]. Here, a change from nematic to isotrope was observed at a temperature up to 70°C depending on the used polymer. By depositing the polymer on a smooth substrate, a change in θ_w of only 3° was observed, while by depositing rough substrates composed of arrays of cylindrical pillars (3 μm in diameter, 6 μm in height, 1.5 μm in spacing), a change from 127 to 86° was measured.

Various inorganic materials also showed thermal response. Shirtcliffe et al. studied the wettability of porous SiO_2 foams obtained by sol-gel from methyltriethoxysilane (MTEOS) [172, 173]. The resulting materials displayed switchable wettability from superhydrophobic to superhydrophilic (Cassie-Baxter-to-Wenzel transition) when they are heated at 400°C. To become hydrophilic, the surface must become more polar. The authors think that this could occur by the formation of new groups or by a change in the relative abundances of apolar methyl groups and polar silica species. Sol-gel foams were also prepared using varying proportions of phenyltriethoxysilane (PhTEOS) and TEOS. The temperatures at which switching occurred were increased when larger fractions of PhTEOS and reversely. SiO_2 suspensions, made from SiO_2 nanoparticles hydrophobically modified with chlorotrimethylsilane and PDMS vinyl terminated, were deposited by spraying [174]. The resulting substrate could reversely switch from superhydrophobic to hydrophobic after cooling at very low temperature (−15°C). Here, the authors attributed this possibility to water vapor condensation on the surface. When the subfreezing film was placed in ambient environment, the humidity in the air condensed to the subfreezing surfaces and increased the surface hydrophilicity. Otherwise, inorganic materials could also be coated using a hydrophobic material in order to achieve superhydrophobic properties [175–179]. Here, the heat treatment could induce the desorption of the hydrophobic material and switch the surface from superhydrophobic to superhydrophilic. However, these kind of materials are reversible but only after surface remodification with the hydrophobic material.

3.3. pH

Materials containing functional acid or basic groups such as amines or carboxylic acids can be used to induce switchable properties by pH changing [180, 181]. For example, at low pH, the COOH group is protonated, while at high, pH it is deprotonated (COO^-) with a much higher hydrophilicity [182]. Zhang et al. modified rough gold substrates with micro/nanostructures by self-assembly of different thiols. They used the dendron thiol 2-(11-mercaptoundecanamido)benzoic acid (MUABA) [183] or mixed solution of $HS(CH_2)_9CH_3$ and $HS(CH_2)_{10}COOH$ [184].

Depending on the surface roughness and the pH, it was possible to obtain switchable surface from superhydrophobic to superhydrophilic. Using mixed solution of $HS(CH_2)_9CH_3$ and $HS(CH_2)_{10}COOH$, the wetting properties were highly dependent on the percentage of each constituent [185, 186]. Using 40 mol% of $HS(CH_2)_{10}COOH$, the surface could change from superhydrophobic ($\theta_w = 154°$) to superhydrophilic ($\theta_w \approx 0°$) as the pH increases.

Mixed solution of $HS(CH_2)_9CH_3$ and $HS(CH_2)_{10}COOH$ was also used on rough mesh substrates [187–191]. $Cu(OH)_2$ nanoneedles were grown on copper meshes by anodization in KOH solution or by immersion in $(NH_4)_2S_2O_8$ and NaOH (**Figure 19**) [187–189]. After surface modification with mixed solution of $HS(CH_2)_9CH_3$ and $HS(CH_2)_{10}COOH$, the best properties were obtained with 60 mol% of $HS(CH_2)_{10}COOH$. The best properties were also obtained for a mesh pore size of 58 μm. Indeed, the authors showed that the pressure that the meshes can support is depending on the mesh geometry and pore size, formation of surface structures on the meshes (nanoneedles) and the surface energy, which here changes with the pH [187–190]. For acidic and neutral water, the meshes were superhydrophobic and underwater superoleophilic. For basic water, the meshes were superhydrophilic and underwater superoleophobic. Here, both the immiscible oil/water mixture and oil-in-water emulsions could be separated on-demand through changing the water pH and with high efficiency and high flux. pH-responsive fabrics were also reported after growth of Ag structures and surface modification with mixed solution of $HS(CH_2)_9CH_3$ and $HS(CH_2)_{10}COOH$ [192].

The change of wettability of DNA nanodevices was also studied [193]. DNA molecules modified with fluorinated hydrophobic groups were fixed to gold substrates by SAM. The conformation of the DNA molecules on the substrate could change with the pH. The substrate was superhydrophilic at low pH and superhydrophobic at high pH.

Various polymers with pH-sensitive groups were also used in the literature. Polymers with carboxylic groups were reported [194–199]. In 2006, Jiang et al. deposited colloidal crystal films made of poly-(styrene-methyl methacrylate-acrylic acid) via a batch emulsion polymerization in the presence of sodium dodecylbenzenesulfonate (SDBS) (**Figure 20**) [194]. At pH 6, the carboxylic groups are in the protonated state (COOH), which could do hydrogen bonds with the SO_3^- groups of SDBS. As a consequence, the hydrophobic tails of the SDBS

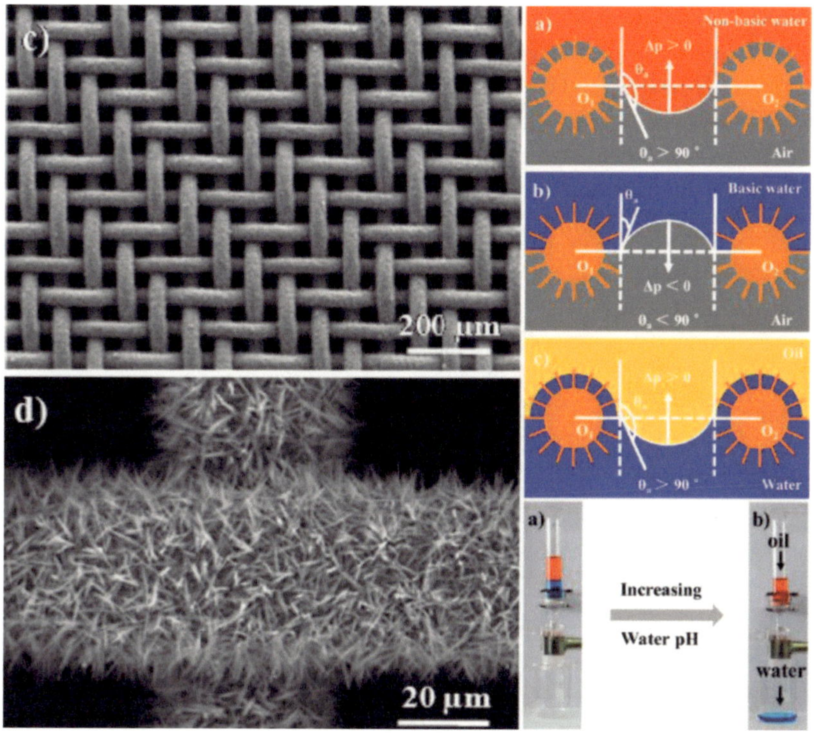

Figure 19. $Cu(OH)_2$ nanoneedles grown on copper steel meshes. The resulting meshes could switch from superhydrophobic and underwater superoleophilic to superhydrophilic and underwater superoleophobic by changing the pH. Ref. [188], Copyright 2015. Reprinted with permission from American Chemical Society, USA.

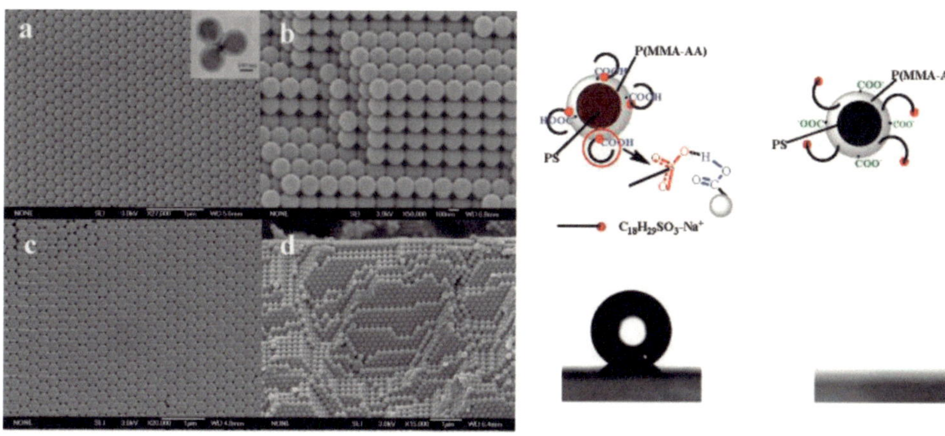

Figure 20. Reversible change from superhydrophobic to superhydrophilic of colloidal crystals (Panels A–D) made of polymers with COOH groups as a function of the pH (Figure on the right). Ref. [194], Copyright 2006. Reprinted with permission from American Chemical Society, USA.

are spread toward air and the surface was superhydrophobic (θ_w = 150.4°). At high pH (pH = 12), the COOH groups are deprotonated (COO^-) suppressing the hydrogen bonds. Here, the surface was superhydrophilic due to the presence of both COO^- and SO_3^-.

Orthophosphoric acids ($ROPO_3H_2$) were also studied. These acids are diacids with a pKa1 between 1 and 2 and a pKa2 between 6 and 7 (**Figure 21**). Three different acids are present dependent on the pH [200–202]. Poly(methacryloyl ethylene phosphate) (PMEP) brushes were used. At pH > 8, the phosphate groups are deprotonated and the electrostatic repulsions between the charged polymer chains led to a swollen state with high hydrophobicity, while at pH < 2, the brushes are protonated and in a collapsed state.

In order to induce basicity, amino groups were also highly used in the literature using different strategies [203–205]. Liu et al. used a triblock copolymer: one block with a hydrophobic group, one block with a pH-sensitive amino group and another one with a functional group for grafting on SiO_2 nanoparticles [203]. The material could be dip-coated on different substrates such as cotton fabric, filter paper and PU foam and could be used for pH-responsive oil/water separation membranes. Among the basic groups, pyridine was also reported. Wang et al. reported the grafting of block copolymer brushes of poly(4-vinylpyridine-*block*-dimethylsiloxane) (P4PV-*b*-PDMS) on SiO_2 nanoparticles [206]. After casting the suspension particles on non-woven cellulose textiles and PU sponges, the resulting materials displayed superhydrophobic and underwater superoleophilic properties at pH 6.5, and superhydrophilic and underwater superoleophobic properties at pH 2.0. Such materials could also be used for controlling the separation of oil/water mixtures by changing the pH. Graphene foams with switchable oil wettability were also reported by grafting block copolymer brushes of poly(2-vinylpyridine-*block*-hexadecyl acrylate) (P2PV-*b*-PHA) [207]. By contrast, other authors chose to graft the polymer directly on substrates [208, 209].

Luo et al. also reported the fabrication of fiber membrane by electrospinning of the block copolymer poly(4-vinylpyridine-*block*-methyl methacrylate) (P4PV-*b*-PMMA) on stainless steel meshes (**Figure 22**) [210]. Using oil/water mixtures, oils can selectively pass through the membrane at pH 3, while at pH 7, water pass selectively. Finally, other authors used block copolymers with both acid and amino groups [211, 212]. For example, Zhou et al. showed that using these kind of polymers it is possible to control the slip length of fluids by changing the pH.

3.4. Voltage

The best advantage of using electrical sensitivity as extern stimulus is the rapidity of implementation [213, 214]. Among the most used materials, conducting polymers are extremely interesting because they can exist in different doping states. The neutral dedoped state is uncharged, while the doped states are charged (**Figure 23**). Moreover, in their doped states, conducting polymers incorporated doping agents (most of the time counter-anions) in order to neutralize the charges present inside the polymer backbone.

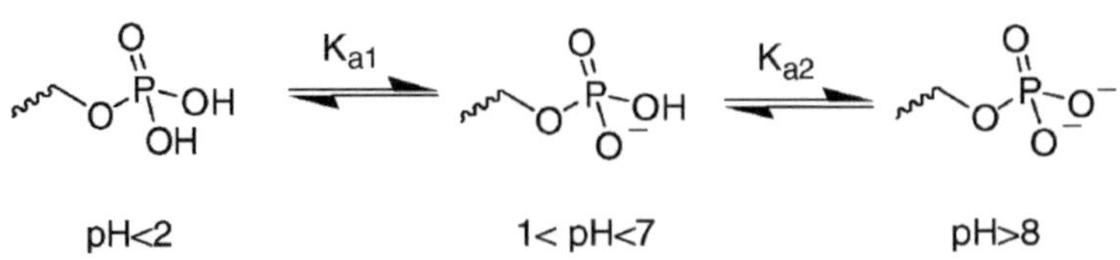

Figure 21. Different species present using orthophosphoric acids as a function of the pH. Ref. [202], Copyright 2005. Reprinted with permission from Royal Society of Chemistry, United Kingdom.

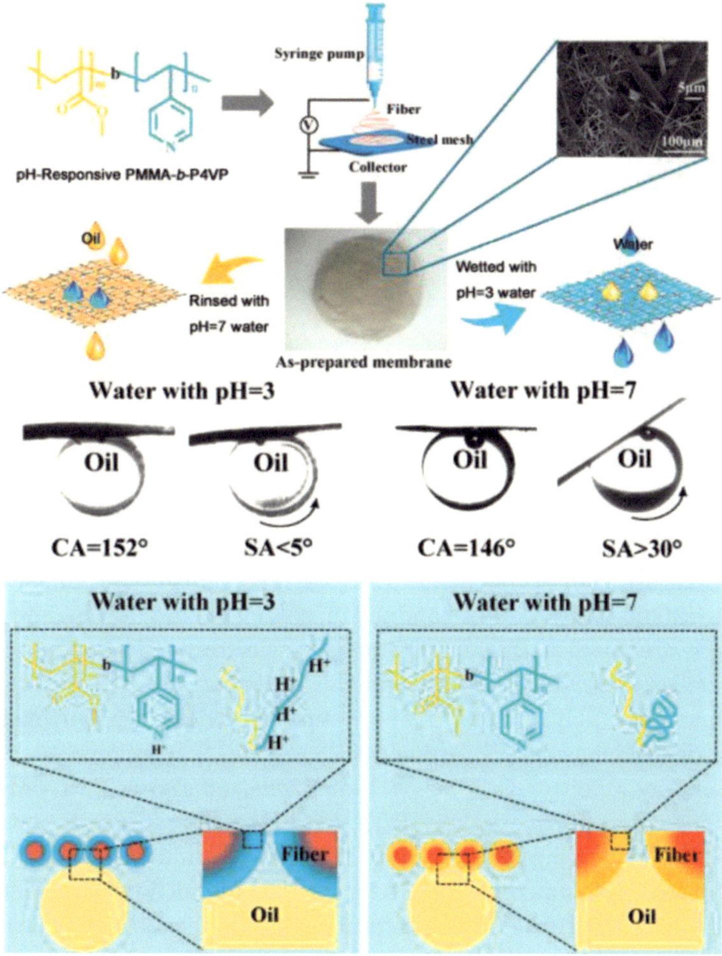

Figure 22. Preparation of pH-induced oil permeation membranes by electrospinning of P4PV-b-PMMA. Ref. [210], Copyright 2015. Reprinted with permission from American Chemical Society, USA.

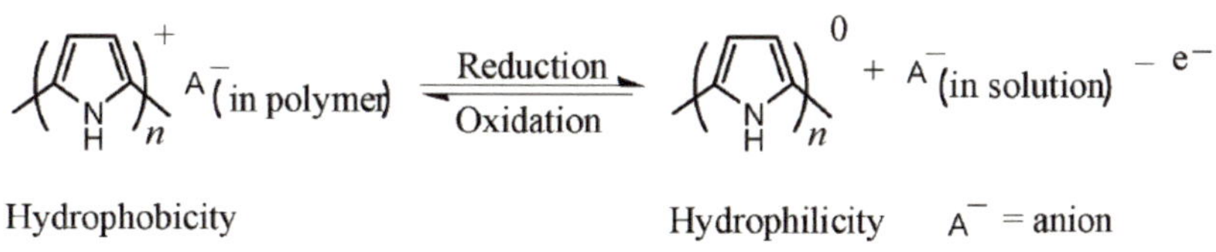

Figure 23. Reversible change in the doping state of conducting polymers by oxidation and reduction [163].

For example, smooth poly(3-alkylthiophene) films prepared by spin coating were studied (**Figure 24**) [215]. In their doping state, different anions (Cl^-, NO_3^-, PO_4^{3-}, CO_3^{2-} and SO_4^{2-}) were introduced. The authors observed that all the anions induced a decrease of θ_w. The highest decrease (from 105.9 to 76.7°) was observed with SO_4^{2-} anions. In order to enhance the wettability difference between the reduced and the oxidized state, the authors also deposited micro-patterned substrates. Then, they observed a much higher decrease from 147.4 to 62.2°.

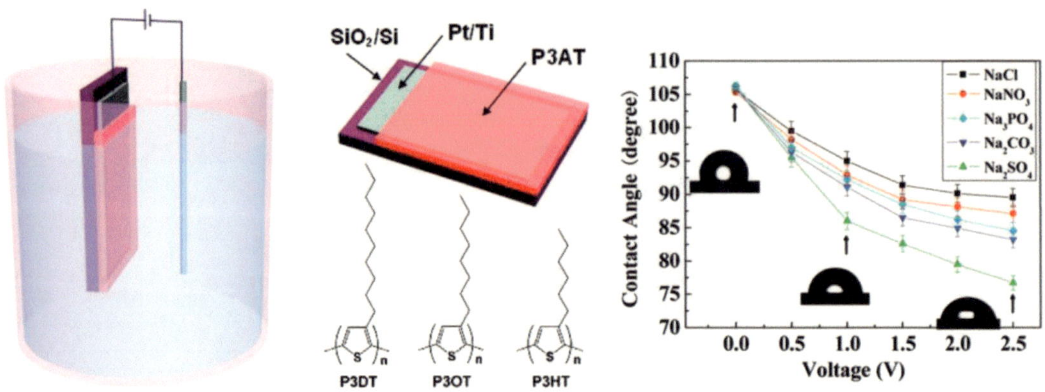

Figure 24. Influence of doping anions in the surface hydrophobicity of smooth poly(3-alkylthiophene). Ref. [215], Copyright 2009. Reprinted with permission from American Chemical Society, USA.

Otherwise, various other techniques can be used to prepare structured conducting polymer films. Among them, using an electrochemical cell, the electropolymerization allows in one step having polymerization, deposition of conducting polymer film and obtaining of structured films. The surface structures are highly dependent on electrochemical parameters (deposition method, time, solvent, electrolyte…) and on the monomer used [216–222]. For example, superhydrophobic rough polypyrrole films were reported by electropolymerization of pyrrole by galvanostatic deposition (constant current of 0.25 mA cm^{-2}) in the presence of highly hydrophobic perfluorooctanesulfonate ($C_8F_{17}SO_3^-$) doping ions and also $FeCl_3$ in order to induce by polymerization and electropolymerization [162]. Here, the surface structures consisted in submicron particles (1–3 μm) forming a porous film. The surface could easily and reversibly switch from superhydrophobic to superhydrophilic by oxidation/reduction using different voltages. Moreover, Chang et al. reported a faster electrical process (3 s) and also eliminated the need to immerse the substrate within an electrolyte [165]. Jiang et al. also reported that the oil adhesion can also be controlled during the doping/dedoping process [222].

Other monomers were also studied [223–228]. Yan et al. reported the use of aniline to produce helical polyaniline fibers in aqueous electrolyte and in the presence of perfluorooctanesulfonic acid by galvanostatic deposition (constant current of 0.2 mA cm^{-2}) [223]. Polyaniline is an interesting polymer because different chemical forms can be produced also depending on the pH. In the presence of tetraethylammonium perfluorooctanesulfonate, the authors reported the possible switching from superhydrophobic (emeraldine salt form) to superhydrophilic (leucoemeraldine base form) by changing the voltage. Poly(3,4-ethylenedioxythiophene) (PEDOT) was also used (**Figure 25**) [224]. Here, two different fluorinated electrolytes were chosen: tetrabutylammonium nonafluorobutanesulfonate ($Bu_4NC_4F_9SO_3$) and tetrabutylammonium heptadecafluorooctanesulfonate ($Bu_4NC_8F_17SO_3$). Their electropolymerization was performed in acetonitrile and at constant potential. Porous films were obtained and the surface morphology was highly dependent on the electrolyte. Superhydrophobic properties were obtained with $Bu_4NC_8F_{17}SO_3$ and using a deposition charge (Qs) of 300 mC cm^{-2} [226, 227]. Lu prepared first a porous PEDOT film on which a second was electrodeposited by cyclic

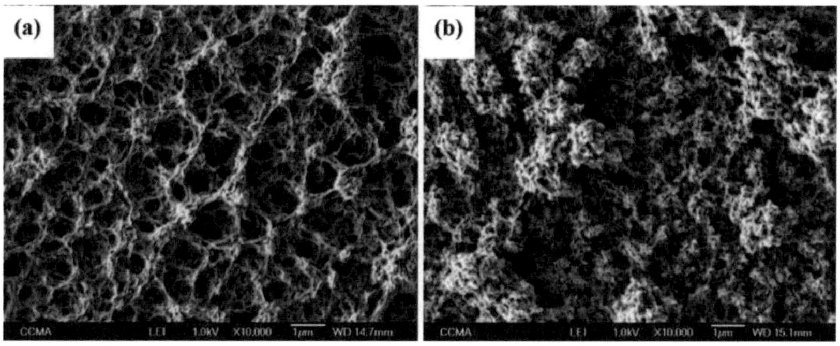

Figure 25. Rough PEDOT substrates obtained in the presence of (a) $Bu_4NC_4F_9SO_3$ and (b) $Bu_4NC_8F_{17}SO_3$ [224].

voltammetry. Using poly(3-methylthiophene), a switchable and reversible surface from superhydrophobic to superhydrophilic was obtained after doping/dedoping in the presence of ClO_4^- anions [170]. By contrast, using poly(3-hexylthiophene), the surface could switch from superhydrophobic to parahydrophobic (high water adhesion) [227]. The surfaces could also induce switchable cell adsorption [228].

Advincula created first polystyrene colloidal crystals in hexagonal packing, on which a polythiophene film with short alkyl chains was electrodeposited by cyclic voltammetry [229]. The surface could switch from superhydrophobic to highly hydrophilic. Here also, the protein and bacterial cell adsorption could also be switched at the same time [230].

Otherwise, different strategies were employed to create nanostructured conducting polymers in solution. For that, polyaniline is a choice material due to the presence of amine groups that allow to induce self-assembly by hydrogen bonds [231–237]. Jiang et al. reported the polymerization *in-situ* on fabrics in the presence of perfluorosebacic acid (HOOC-C_8F_{16}-COOH) and $FeCl_3$, as dopant and oxidant, respectively [232]. Nanoparticles were formed on the fabrics. The resulting fabrics could switch from superhydrophobic to superhydrophilic by doping/dedoping while the dedoping could be performed in the presence of NH_3 gas. Fabrics with switchable wettability from superoleophobic to superoleophilic were also reported using perfluorooctanoic acid [233, 234]. In order to prepare membranes with selective responsivity for oil/water separation, stainless steel meshes were coated with root-like polyaniline nanofibers fabricated by emulsion polymerization [235]. The meshes could switch from superhydrophobic to superhydrophilic at different voltages.

Metal ions and organic molecules sensitive to redox reactions can also be used to switch the surface wettability by voltage [238, 239]. For example, Ag + −biphenyldithiol (BPDT) SAMS could be converted to Ag^0-BPDT by applying a difference potential [238]. Ferricyanide ($[Fe(CN)_6]^{3-}$) could also be converted into $[Fe(CN)_6]^{4-}$ [240]. Huck et al. showed that polycationic [2-(methacryloyloxy)-trimethylammonium chloride] (PMETAC) brushes coordinated to $[Fe(CN)_6]^{3-}$ had $\theta_w = 41–44°$ while the brushes coordinated to $[Fe(CN)_6]^{4-}$ had $\theta_w = 26–27°$ [241].

The reorientation of polyelectrolyte conformation is another phenomenon induced by electric potential [242, 243]. Choi et al. observed that a SAM of (16-mercapto)hexadecanoic acid

(MHA) deposited on a gold substrate could undergo a transition from a straight conformation to a curved one by applying an electric potential. The molecules in the straight conformation are hydrophilic due to the presence of carboxylate ions and that in the curved conformation are hydrophobic due to the presence of the hydrophobic chains.

Electrowetting is another method allowing the control of the surface wettability by applying an extern electric field. In this process, a water droplet is placed on a superhydrophobic surfaces coated with an insulating layer. The applying of the electric field induces an accumulation of charges and decreases the solid-liquid interface (γ_{SL}) and as a consequence the surface hydrophobicity, as shown in **Figure 26** [244, 245].

In 2004, Krupenkin et al. studied the electrowetting of superhydrophobic substrates prepared by modifying nanostructured silicon substrates with a low surface energy material [246]. After electrowetting, they could change the surface wettability from superhydrophobic to superhydrophilic. Vertically aligned superhydrophobic carbon nanofibers and ZnO nanorods

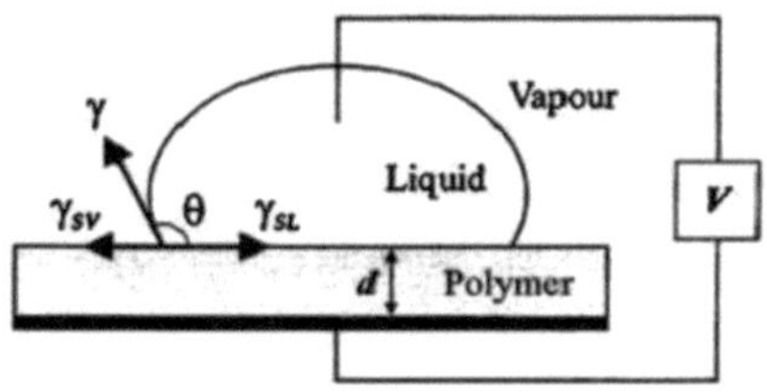

Figure 26. Schematic representation of electrowetting experiment. Ref. [244], Copyright 2003. Reprinted with permission from American Chemical Society, USA.

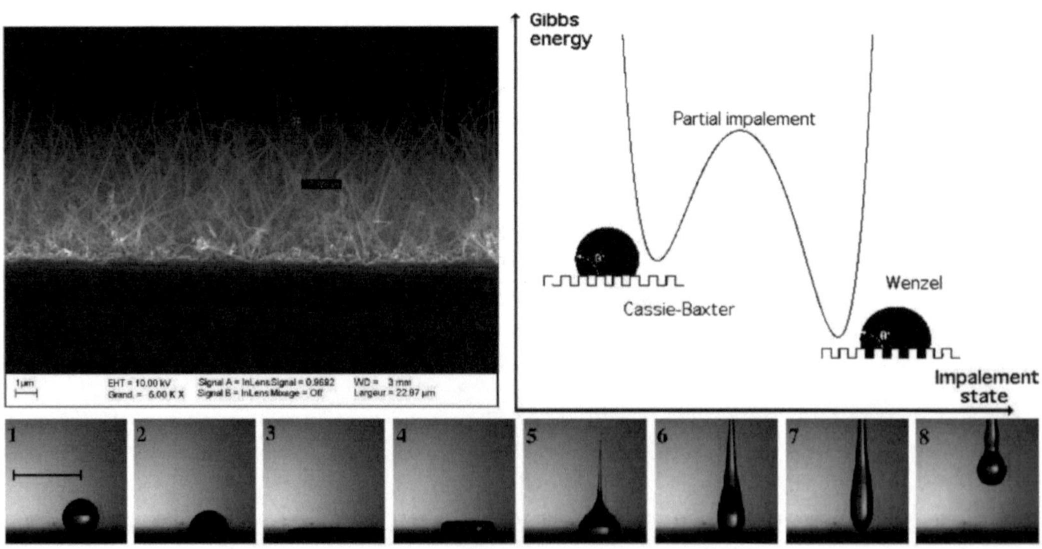

Figure 27. Relationship between the resistance to drop impact impalement and electrowetting impalement using silicon nanowires with double nanotextures. Ref. [254], Copyright 2008. Reprinted with permission from American Chemical Society, USA.

were also highly used in the literature to induce a switch from superhydrophobic to hydrophilic or superhydrophilic [247–251]. Boukherroub et al. reported the possible obtaining of reversible electrowetting on silicon nanowires with double nanotextures (length of 10 and 30 μm) [252–255]. They found a relationship between the resistance to drop impact impalement and electrowetting impalement (**Figure 27**) [254]. The thresholds for drop impact and electrowetting irreversibility increase and the contact angle hysteresis decrease when the length and the density of nanowires increase. Other mechanisms for reversible electrowetting were also reported in the literature [256, 257]. Otherwise, electrowetting could also be used to control protein adsorption or for accelerating reaction by mixing liquid droplets [258, 259].

Author details

Sabri Taleb, Thierry Darmanin* and Frédéric Guittard

*Address all correspondence to: thierry.darmanin@unice.fr

Université Côte d'Azur, NICE Lab, IMREDD, Nice, France

References

[1] Darmanin T, Guittard F. Materials Today. 2015;**18**:273-285

[2] Barthlott B, Neinhuis C. Planta. 1997;**202**:1-8

[3] Liu Y, Li G. Journal of Colloid and Interface Science. 2012;**388**:235-242

[4] Wang WK, Zheng ML, Chen WQ, Jin F, Cao YY, Zhao ZS, Duan XM. Langmuir. 2011; **27**:3249-3253

[5] Mele E, Girardo S, Pisignano D. Langmuir. 2012;**28**:5312-5317

[6] Bush JWM, Hu DL, Prakash M. Advances in Insect Physiology. 2007;**34**:117-192

[7] Sun M, Watson GS, Zheng Y, Watson JA, Liang A. Journal of Experimental Biology. 2009;**212**:3148-3155

[8] Hensel R, Helbig R, Aland S, Braun HG, Voigt A, Neinhuis C, Werner C. Langmuir. 2013; **29**:1100-1112

[9] Feng L, Zhang Y, Xi J, Zhu Y, Wang N, Xia F, Jiang L. Langmuir. 2008;**24**:4114-4119

[10] Autumn K. Journal of Experimental Biology. 2006;**209**:3558-3568

[11] Bixler GD, Bhushan B. Nanoscale. 2014;**6**:76-96

[12] Pinchasik BE, Steinkühler J, Wuytens P, Skirtach AG, Fratzl P, Möhwald H. Langmuir. 2015;**31**:13734-13742

[13] Zeng H, Pesika N, Tian Y, Zhao B, Chen Y, Tirrell M, Turner KL, Israelachvili JN. Langmuir. 2009;**25**:7486-7495

[14] Liu F, Lu R, Pan QACS. Sustainable Chemistry and Engineering. 2017;**5**:922-928

[15] Young T. Philosophical Transactions of the Royal Society of London. 1805;**95**:65-87

[16] Wenzel RN. Industrial and Engineering Chemistry. 1936;**28**:988-994

[17] Cassie ABD, Baxter S. Transactions of the Faraday Society. 1944;**40**:546-551

[18] Su Y, Ji B, Zhang K, Gao H, Huang Y, Hwang K. Langmuir. 2010;**26**:4984-4989

[19] Yu Y, Zhao ZH, Zheng QS. Langmuir. 2007;**23**:8212-8216

[20] Bellanger H, Darmanin T, Taffin de Givenchy E, Guittard F. Chemical Reviews. 2014; **114**:2694-2716

[21] Liu T, Kim CJ. Science. 2014;**346**:1096-1100

[22] Tuteja A, Choi W, Ma M, Mabry JM, Mazzella SA, Rutledge GC, McKinley GH, Cohen RE. Science. 2007;**318**:1618-1622

[23] Marmur A. Soft Matter. 2012;**8**:6867-6870

[24] Verho T, Korhonen JT, Sainiemi L, Jokinen V, Bower C, Franze K, Franssila S, Andrew P, Ikkala O, RHA R. Proceedings of the National Academy of Sciences U.S.A. 2012;**109**: 10210-10213

[25] Boreyko JB, Collier CP. Journal of Physical Chemistry C. 2013;**117**:18084-18090

[26] Wang S, Song Y, Jiang L. Journal of Photochemistry and Photobiology C. 2007;**8**:18-29

[27] Banerjee S, Dionysiou DD, Pillai SC. Applied Catalysis, B. 2015;**176–177**:396-428

[28] Pelaez M, Nolan NT, Pillai SC, Seery MK, Falaras P, Kontos AG, Dunlop PSM, Hamilton JWJ, Byrne JA, O'Shea K, Entezari MH, Dionysiou DD. Applied Catalysis, B. 2012;**125**: 331-349

[29] Wang R, Hashimoto K, Fujishima A, Chikuni M, Kojima E, Kitamura A, Shimohigoshi M, Watanabe T. Nature. 1997;**388**:431-432

[30] Wang R, Hashimoto K, Fujishima A, Chikuni M, Kojima E, Kitamura A, Shimohigoshi M, Watanabe T. Advanced Materials. 1998;**10**:135-138

[31] Sakai N, Wang R, Fujishima A, Watanabe T, Hashimoto K. Langmuir. 1998;**14**:5918-5920

[32] Stevens N, Priest CI, Sedev R, Ralston J. Langmuir. 2003;**19**:3272-3275

[33] Caputo G, Nobile C, Kipp T, Blasi L, Grillo V, Carlino E, Manna L, Cingolani R, Cozzoli PD, Athanassiou A. Journal of Physical Chemistry C. 2008;**112**:701-714

[34] Sakai N, Fujishima A, Watanabe T, Hashimoto K. Journal of Physical Chemistry B. 2003; **107**:1028-1035

[35] Gu Z, Fujishima A, Sato O. Angewandte Chemie, International Edition. 2002;**41**: 2067-2070

[36] Tadanaga K, Morinaga J, Matsuda A, Minami T. Chemistry of Materials. 2000;**12**:590-592

[37] Feng X, Zhai J, Jiang L. Angewandte Chemie, International Edition. 2005;**44**:5115-5118

[38] Wang D, Liu Y, Liu X, Zhou FW, Xue Q. Chemical Communications. 2009:7018-7020

[39] Antony RP, Mathews T, Dash S, Tyagi AK. Journal of Physical Chemistry C. 2013; **117**:6851-6860

[40] Lai Y, Pan F, Xu C, Fuchs H, Chi L. Advanced Materials. 2013;**25**:1682-1686

[41] Sun W, Zhou S, Chen P, Peng L. Chemical Communications. 2008:603-605

[42] Zhang X, Kono H, Liu Z, Nishimoto S, Tryk DA, Murakami T, Sakai H, Abe M, Fujishima A. Chemical Communications. 2007:4949-4951

[43] Zhang X, Jin M, Liu Z, Nishimo S, Saito H, Murakami T, Fujishima A. Langmuir. 2006;**22**:9477-9479

[44] Zhang X, Jin M, Liu Z, Tryk DA, Nishimoto S, Murakami T, Fujishima A. Journal of Physical Chemistry C. 2007;**111**:14521-14529

[45] Yong J, Chen F, Yang Q, Farooq U, Hou X. Journal of Materials Chemistry A. 2015; **3**:10703-10709

[46] Hoshian S, Jokinen V, Hjort K, Ras RHA, Franssila S. ACS Applied Materials and Interfaces. 2015;**7**:15593-15599

[47] Sahoo M, Mathews T, Antony RP, Krishna DN, Dash S, Tyagi AK. ACS Applied Materials and Interfaces. 2013;**5**:3967-3974

[48] Yin Y, Huang R, Zhang W, Zhang M, Wang C. Chemical Engineering Journal. 2016; **289**:99-105

[49] Naghdi S, Jaleh B, Shahbazi N. Applied Surface Science. 2016;**368**:409-416

[50] Stepien M, Saarinen JJ, Teisala H, Tuominen M, Aromaa M, Haapanen J, Kuusipalo J, Makela JM, Toivakka M. Langmuir. 2013;**29**:3780-3790

[51] Qin L, Zhao J, Lei S, Pan Q. ACS Applied Materials and Interfaces. 2014;**6**:21355-21362

[52] Li L, Liu L, Lei J, He J, Li N, Pan F. Journal of Materials Chemistry A. 2016;**4**:12334-12340

[53] Wang Y, Lai C, Wang X, Liu Y, Hu H, Guo Y, Ma K, Fei B, Xin JH. ACS Applied Materials and Interfaces. 2016;**8**:25612-25620

[54] Kim DH, Jung MC, Cho SH, Kim SH, Kim HY, Lee HJ, KH O, Moon MW. Scientific Reports. 2015;**5**:12908

[55] Sun RD, Nakajima A, Watanabe T, Hashimoto K. Journal of Physical Chemistry B. 2001; **105**:1984-1990

[56] Miyauchi M, Shimai A, Tsuru Y. Journal of Physical Chemistry B. 2005;**109**:13307-13311

[57] Feng X, Feng L, Jin M, Zhai J, Jiang L, Zhu D. Journal of American Chemical Society. 2004;**126**:62-63

[58] Mondal C, Ganguly M, Sinha AK, Pal J, Pal T. RSC Advances. 2013;**3**:5937-5944

[59] Xue X, Zhang Z, Men X, Yang J, Xu X. Applied Surface Science. 2010;**256**:7619-7922

[60] Park J, Lee S, Lee J, Yong K. Advanced Materials. 2013;**25**:6423-6429

[61] Tian D, Zhang X, Tian Y, Wu Y, Wang X, Zhai J, Jiang L. Journal of Materials Chemistry. 2012;**22**:19652-19657

[62] H L ZM, Liu S, Ma L, Zhu C, Xiong Z. Surface and Coatings Technology. 2013;**224**:88-92

[63] Nakate UT, Patil P, Bulakhe RN, Lokhande CD, Kale SN, Naushad M, Mane RS. Journal of Colloid and Interface Science. 2016;**480**:109-117

[64] Li J, Jing Z, Yang Y, Zha F, Yan L, Lei Z. Applied Surface Science. 2014;**289**:1-5

[65] Ennaceri H, Wang L, Erfurt D, Riedel W, Mangalgiri G, Khaldoun A, El Kenz A, Benyoussef A, Ennaoui A. Surface and Coatings Technology. 2016;**299**:169-176

[66] Qing Y, Yang C, Yu Z, Zhang Z, Hu Q, Liu C. Journal of Electrochemical Society. 2016;**163**:D385-D391

[67] Li M, Zhai J, Liu H, Song Y, Jiang L, Zhu D. Journal of Physical Chemistry B. 2003; **107**:9954-9957

[68] Zhang X, Sato O, Fujishima A. Langmuir. 2004;**20**:6065-6067

[69] Liu H, Feng L, Zhai J, Jiang L, Zhu D. Langmuir. 2004;**20**:5659-5661

[70] Shaik UP, Kshirsagar S, Krishna MG, Tewari SP, Purkayastha DD, Madhurima V. Materials Letters. 2012;**75**:51-53

[71] Laurenti M, Verna A, Fontana M, Stassi S, Canavese G, Marasso SL, Cauda V. Advanced Materials Interfaces. 2016;**3**:1600110/1-1600110/X

[72] Li J, Sun Q, Han S, Wang J, Wang Z, Jin C. Progress in Organic Coatings. 2015;**87**:155-160

[73] Zhang B, Lu S, Xu W, Cheng Y. Applied Surface Science. 2016;**360**:904-914

[74] Shaik UP, Purkayastha DD, Krishna MG, Madhurima V. Applied Surface Science. 2015;**330**:292-299

[75] Wood TJ, Hurst GA, Schofield WCE, Thompson RL, Oswald G, Evans JSO, Sharples GJ, Pearson C, Perry MC, Badyal JPS. Journal of Materials Chemistry. 2012;**22**:3859-3867

[76] Mondal C, Sinha AK, Ganguly M, Pal J, Dhara S, Negishi Y, Pal T. CrystEngComm. 2014;**16**:4322-4328

[77] Yong J, Chen F, Yang Q, Fang Y, Huo J, Hou X. Chemical Communications. 2015;**51**:9813-9816

[78] Papadopoulou EL, Barberoglou M, Zorba V, Manousaki A, Pagkozidis A, Stratakis E, Fotakis C. Journal of Physical Chemistry C. 2009;**113**:2891-2895

[79] Frysali MA, Papoutsakis L, Kenanakis G, Anastasiadis SH. Journal of Physical Chemistry C. 2015;**119**:25401-25407

[80] Wang S, Feng X, Yao J, Jiang L. Angewandte Chemie, International Edition. 2006;**45**: 1264-1267

[81] Jiang T, Guo Z. Applied Surface Science. 2016;**387**:412-418

[82] Lim HS, Kwak D, Lee DY, Lee SG, Cho K. Journal of American Chemical Society. 2007;**129**:4128-4129

[83] Zhu W, Feng X, Feng L, Jiang L. Chemical Communications. 2006:2753

[84] Pan J, Song X, Zhang J, Shen H, Xiong Q. Journal of Physical Chemistry C. 2011;**115**: 22225-22231

[85] Pei MD, Wang B, Li E, Zhang X, Xm S, Yan H. Applied Surface Science. 2010;**256**:5824-5827

[86] Cui H, Yang GZ, Sun Y, Wang CX. Applied Physics Letters. 2010;**97**:183112/1-183112/3

[87] Zhong M, Zheng M, Zeng A, Ma L. Applied Physics Letters. 2008;**92**:093118/1-093118/3

[88] Chang YH, Hau NY, Liu C, Huang YT, Li CC, Shih K, Feng SP. Nanoscale. 2014;**6**:15309-15315

[89] Xu P, Wang F, Yang C, Ou J, Li W, Amirfazli A. Surface and Coatings Technology. 2016; **294**:47-53

[90] Kietzig AM, Hatzikiriakos SG, Englezos P. Langmuir. 2009;**25**:4821-4827

[91] Yan B, Tao J, Pang C, Zheng Z, Shen Z, Huan C, Yu T. Langmuir. 2008;**24**:10569-10571

[92] Li J, Han Q, Zhang Y, Zhang W, Dong M, Besenbacher F, Yang R, Wang C. ACS Applied Materials and Interfaces. 2013;**5**:9816-9822

[93] Kwak G, Lee M, Yong K. Langmuir. 2010;**26**:9964-9967

[94] Gu C, Zhang J, Tu J. Journal of Colloid and Interface Science. 2010;**352**:573-579

[95] Su R, Liu H, Kong T, Song Q, Li N, Jin G, Cheng G. Langmuir. 2011;**27**:13220-13325

[96] Su C, Lu Z, Zhao H, Yang H, Chen R. Applied Surface Science. 2015;**353**:735-743

[97] Chen Y, Li X, Glasper MJ, Liu L, Chung HJ, Nychka JA. RSC Advances. 2016;**6**:92833-92838

[98] Yang J, Zhang Z, Men X, Xu X, Zhu X. Langmuir. 2010;**26**:10198-10202

[99] Li J, Ling J, Yan L, Wang Q, Zha F, Lei Z. Surface and Coatings Technology. 2014;**258**: 142-145

[100] Wang HZ, Huang ZP, Cai QJ, Kulkarni K, Chen C-L, Carnahan D, Ren ZF. Carbon. 2010;**48**:868-875

[101] Huang Y, Chen X, Zhang MQ. Journal of Materials Science. 2014;**49**:3025-3033

[102] Kwon Y, Weon BM, Won KH, Je JH, Hwu Y, Margaritono G. Langmuir. 2009;**25**:1927-1929

[103] Hou W, Wang Q. Langmuir. 2009;**25**:6875-6879

[104] Pant R, Singha S, Bandyopadhyay A, Khare K. Applied Surface Science. 2014;**292**:777-781

[105] Xue X, Zhang Z, Guo F, Yang J, Zhu X. Applied Surface Science. 2011;**57**:7054-7060

[106] Xu QF, Liu Y, Lin FJ, Mondal B, Lyons AM. ACS Applied Materials and Interfaces. 2013;**5**:8915-8924

[107] Zhang W, Lu X, Xin Z, Zhou C, Liu J. RSC Advances. 2015;**5**:55513-55519

[108] Zhang W, Lu X, Xin Z, Zhou C. RSC Advances. 2016;**6**:106054-106063

[109] Wang SF, Kao TH, Cheng CC, Chang CJ, Chen JK. Applied Surface Science. 2015;**357**:1634-1646

[110] Yan L, Li J, Li W, Zha F, Feng H, Hu D. Materials Letters. 2016;**163**:247-249

[111] Deng ZY, Wang W, Mao LH, Wang CF, Chen S. Journal of Materials Chemistry A. 2014;**2**:4178-4184

[112] Qing Y, Yang C, Yu N, Shang Y, Sun Y, Wang L, Liu C. Chemical Engineering Journal. 2016;**290**:37-44

[113] Sawada E, Kakehi H, Chounan Y, Miura M, Sato Y, Isu N, Sawada H. Composites: Part B. 2010;**41**:498-502

[114] Liu Y, Lin Z, Lin W, Moon KS, Wong CP. ACS Applied Materials and Interfaces. 2012;**4**:3959-3964

[115] Delorme N, Bardeau JF, Bulou A, Poncin-Epaillard F. Langmuir. 2005;**21**:12278-12282

[116] Cooper CGF, MacDonald JC, Soto E, McGimpsey WG. Journal of American Chemical Society. 2004;**126**:1032-1033

[117] Driscoll PF, Purohit N, Wanichacheva N, Lambert CR, McGimpsey WG. Langmuir. 2007;**23**:13181-13187

[118] Abbott S, Ralston J, Reynolds G, Hayes R. Langmuir. 1999;**15**:8923-8928

[119] Ichimura K, SK O, Nakagawa M. Science. 2000;**288**:1624-1626

[120] SK O, Nakagawa M, Ichimura K. Journal of Materials Chemistry. 2002;**12**:2262-2269

[121] Jiang W, Wang G, He Y, Wang X, An Y, Song Y, Jiang L. Chemical Communications. 2005:3550-3552

[122] Siewierski LM, Brittain WJ, Petrash S, Foster MD. Langmuir. 1996;**12**:5838-5844

[123] Feng C, Zhang Y, Jin J, Song Y, Xie L, Qu G, Jiang LD, Zhu D. Langmuir. 2001;**17**:4593-4597

[124] Lim HS, Han JT, Kwak D, Jin M, Cho K. Journal of American Chemical Society. 2006;**128**:14458-14559

[125] Prescher D, Thiele T, Ruhmann R, Schulz G. Journal of Fluorine Chemistry. 1995;**74**: 185-189

[126] Pan S, Guo R, Xu W. Soft Matter. 2014;**10**:9187-9192

[127] Jin C, Yan R, Huang J. Journal of Materials Chemistry. 2011;**21**:17519-17525

[128] Huang J, Huang Y, He C, Gao Y. RSC Advances. 2015;**5**:100339-100346

[129] Chen L, He C, Huang Y, Huang J, Zhang Y, Gao Y. Applied Polymer Science. 2016; **133**:43540/1-43540/9

[130] Pang X, Pan S, Feng S, Chen H, Li L, Su X, Xiong Y, Xu W. Macromolecular Materials and Engineering. 2012;**297**:979-984

[131] Zhang J, Zhang W, Zhou N, Weng Y, Hu Z. RSC Advances. 2014;**4**:24973-24977

[132] Li C, Cheng F, Lv J, Zhao Y, Liu M, Jiang L, Yu Y. Soft Matter. 2012;**8**:3730-3733

[133] Groten J, Bunte CJ, Ruehe J. Langmuir. 2012;**28**:15038-15046

[134] Li C, Zhang Y, Ju J, Cheng F, Liu M, Jiang LY, Yu Y. Advanced Functional Materials. 2012;**22**:760-763

[135] Liu X, Cai M, Liang Y, Zhou F, Liu W. Soft Matter. 2011;**7**:3331-3336

[136] Uchida K, Izumi N, Sukata S, Kojima Y, Nakamura S, Irie M. Angewandte Chemie, International Edition. 2006;**45**:6470-6473

[137] Nishikawa N, Uyama A, Kamitanaka T, Mayama H, Kojima Y, Yokojima S, Nakamura S, Tsujii K, Uchida K. Chemistry – An Asian Journal. 2011;**6**:2400-2406

[138] Uyama A, Yamazoe S, Shigematsu S, Morimoto M, Yokojima S, Mayama H, Kojima Y, Nakamura S, Irie M, Uchida K. Langmuir. 2011;**27**:6395-6400

[139] Nishikawa N, Kiyohara H, Sakiyama S, Yamazoe S, Mayama H, Tsujioka T, Kojima Y, Yokojima S, Nakamura S, Uchida K. Langmuir. 2012;**28**:17817-17824

[140] Nishikawa N, Sakiyama S, Yamazoe S, Kojima Y, Ei N, Tsujioka T, Mayama H, Yokojima S, Nakamura S, Uchida K. Langmuir. 2013;**29**:8164-8169

[141] Oropesa-Nunez R, Fragouli D, Pignatelli F, Scarpellini A, Gigliotti E, Samoylova E, Athanassiou A. Langmuir. 2014;**30**:13058-13064

[142] Rosario R, Gust D, Hayes M, Jahnke F, Springer J, Garcia AA. Langmuir. 2002;**18**:8062-8069

[143] Hayashida S, Sato H, Sugawara S. Polymer Journal. 1986;**18**:227-235

[144] Athanassiou A, Lygeraki MI, Pisignano D, Lakiotaki K, Varda M, Mele E, Fotakis C, Cingolani R, Anastasiadis SH. Langmuir. 2006;**22**:2329-2333

[145] Rosario R, Gust D, Garcia AA, Hayes M, Taraci JL, Clement T, Dailey JW, Picraux ST. Journal of Physical Chemistry B. 2004;**108**:12640-12642

[146] Wang D, Jiao P, Wang J, Zhang Q, Feng L, Yang Z. Journal of Applied Polymer Science. 2012;**125**:870-875

[147] Vlassiouk I, Park CD, Vail SA, Gust D, Smirnov S. Nano Letters. 2006;(5):1013-1017

[148] Zhu H, Yang S, Chen D, Li N, Xu Q, Li H, He J, Liu L. Advanced Materials Interfaces. 2015;**3**:1500683/1-1500683/x

[149] Kehrlosser D, Trager J, Kim HC, Hampp N. Langmuir. 2010;**26**:3878-3882

[150] Li L, Pan S, Pang X, Chen H, Hu D, Ke L, Xiong Y, Xu W. Soft Matter. 2012;**8**:7357-7360

[151] Sun TL, Wang GJ, Feng L, Liu BQ, Ma YM, Jiang L, Zhu DB. Angewandte Chemie, International Edition. 2004;**43**:357-360

[152] Wang Y, Lai C, Hu H, Liu Y, Fei B, Xin JH. RSC Advances. 2015;**5**:51078-51085

[153] De Leon A, Advincula RC. ACS Applied Materials and Interfaces. 2014;**6**:22666-22672

[154] Ryu HY, Yoon SH, Han DH, Hafeez H, Paluvai NR, Lee CS, Park JG. Progress in Organic Coatings. 2016;**99**:295-301

[155] Chen H, Pan S, Xiong Y, Peng C, Pang X, Li L, Xiong Y, Xu W. Applied Surface Science. 2012;**258**:9505-9509

[156] Fu Q, Rao GVR, Basame SB, Keller DJ, Artyushkova K, Fulghum JE, Lopez GP. Journal of the American Chemical Society. 2004;**126**:8904-8905

[157] Wang N, Zhao Y, Jiang L. Macromolecular Rapid Communications. 2008;**29**:485-489

[158] SY G, Wang ZM, Li JB, Ren J. Macromolecular Materials and Engineering. 2010;**295**:32-36

[159] Muthiah P, Boyle TJ, Sigmund W. Macromolecular Materials and Engineering. 2013; **298**:1251-1258

[160] Muthiah P, Hoppe SM, Boyle TJ, Sigmund W. Macromolecular Materials and Engineering. 2011;**32**:1716-1721

[161] Song W. Nanoscale. 2014;**6**:13435-13439

[162] Ou R, Wei J, Jiang L, Simon GP, Wang H. Environmental Science and Technology. 2016; **50**:906-914

[163] Yang H, Zhu H, Hendrix MMRM, Lousberg NJHGM, de With G, Esteves ACC, Xin JJ. Advanced Materials. 2013;**25**:1150-1154

[164] Chunder A, Etcheverry K, Londe G, Cho HJ, Zhai L. Colloids and Surfaces, A. 2009; **333**:187-193

[165] Londe G, Chunder A, Wesser A, Zhai L, Cho HJ. Sensors and Actuators B. 2008;**132**:431-438

[166] Chen Y, Gai P, Xue J, Zhang JR, Zhu JJ. Biosensors and Bioelectronics. 2015;**74**:142-149

[167] Hu S, Cao X, Song Y, Li C, Xie P, Jiang L. Chemical Communications. 2008:2025-2027

[168] Gao Z, Zhai X, Wang C. Applied Surface Science. 2015;**359**:209-214

[169] Wang CF, Liao CS, Kuo SW, Lin HC. Applied Surface Science. 2011;**257**:9152-9157

[170] Li C, Guo R, Jiang X, Hu S, Li L, Cao X, Yang H, Song Y, Ma Y, Jiang L. Advanced Materials. 2009;**21**:4254-4258

[171] ZL W, Buguin A, Yang H, Taulemesse JM, Le Moigne N, Bergeret A, Wang X, Keller P. Advanced Materials. 2013;**23**:3070-3076

[172] Shirtcliffe NJ, McHale G, Newton MI, Perry CC, Roach P. Chemical Communications. 2005:3135-3137

[173] Mahadik SA, Mahadik DB, Parale VG, Wagh PB, Gupta S, Rao AV. Journal of Sol-Gel Science and Technology. 2012;**62**:490-494

[174] Zhang X, Guo Y, Zhang P, Wu Z, Zhang Z. ACS Applied Materials and Interfaces. 2012; **4**:1742-1746

[175] Shi Y, Yang W, Bai J, Feng X, Wang Y. Surface and Coatings Technology. 2014;**253**:148-153

[176] Shi Y, Yang W, Feng X, Feng L, Yue G, Wang Y. RSC Advances. 2015;**5**:26107-26113

[177] Wang Z, Zhu L, Li W, Liu H. ACS Applied Materials and Interfaces. 2013;**5**:4808-4814

[178] Liang W, Liu Y, Sun H, Zhu Z, Zhao X, Li A, Deng W. RSC Advances. 2014;**4**:12590-12595

[179] Liang W, Zhu L, Li W, Liu H. RSC Advances. 2015;**5**:38100-38110

[180] Khopade AJ, Caruso F. Langmuir. 2002;**18**:7669-7676

[181] Holmes-Farley SR, Bain CD, Whitesides GM. Langmuir. 1988;**4**:921-931

[182] Wilson MD, Whitesides GM. Journal of the American Chemical Society. 1988;**110**:8718-8719

[183] Jiang Y, Wang Z, Yu X, Shi F, Xu H, Zhang X. Langmuir. 2005;**21**:1986-1990

[184] Yu X, Wang ZQ, Jiang YG, Shi F, Zhang X. Advanced Materials. 2005;**17**:1289-1293

[185] Liu Y, Yao W, Wang G, Wang Y, Moita AS, Han Z, Ren L. Chemical Engineering Journal. 2016;**303**:565-574

[186] Xiao M, Guo X, Cheng M, Ju G, Zhang Y, Shi F. Small. 2014;**10**:859-865

[187] Cheng Z, Du M, Fu K, Zhang N, Sun K. ACS Applied Materials and Interfaces. 2012;**4**:5826-5832

[188] Cheng Z, Wang J, Lai H, Du Y, Hou R, Li C, Zhang N, Sun K. Langmuir. 2015;**31**:1393-1399

[189] Cheng Z, Li C, Lai H, Du Y, Liu H, Liu M, Jin L, Zhang C, Zhang SK. RSC Advances. 2016;**6**:72317-72325

[190] Tie L, Guo Z, Liu W. Langmuir. 2015;**7**:10641-10649

[191] Wang B, Guo Z. Chemical Communications. 2013;**49**:9416-9418

[192] Wang B, Guo Z, Liu W. RSC Advances. 2014;**4**:14684-14690

[193] Wang S, Liu H, Liu D, Ma X, Fang X, Jiang L. Angewandte Chemie, International Edition. 2007;**46**:3915-3917

[194] Wang J, Hu J, Wen Y, Song Y, Jiang L. Chemistry of Materials. 2006;**18**:4984-4986

[195] Kim BY, Bruening ML. Langmuir. 2003;**19**:94-99

[196] Connal LA, Li Q, Quinn JF, Tjipto E, Caruso F, Qiao G. Macromolecules. 2008;**41**:2620-2626

[197] Synytska A, Diez MS, Lonov L. Langmuir. 2007;**23**:5205-5209

[198] Fu Y, Bai SL, Cui S, Qiu D, Wang Z, Zhang X. Macromolecules. 2002;**35**:9451-9458

[199] Zhang H, Fu Y, Wang D, Wang L, Wang Z, Zhang X. Langmuir. 2003;**19**:8497-8502

[200] Zhou F, Shu W, Welland ME, Huck WTS. Journal of the American Chemical Society. 2006;**128**:5326-5327

[201] Dai X, Zhou F, Khan N, Huck WTS, Kaminski CF. Langmuir. 2008;**24**:13182-13185

[202] Zhou F, Huck WTS. Chemical Communications. 2005:5999-6001

[203] Dang Z, Liu L, Li Y, Xiang Y, Guo G. ACS Applied Materials and Interfaces. 2015;**7**: 19643-19650

[204] Karaman M, Cabuk N. Thin Solid Films. 2012;**520**:6484-6488

[205] Mishra S, Ashaduzzaman M, Mishra P, Swart HC, Turner APF, Tiwari A. Biosensors and Bioelectronics. 2017;**89**:305-311

[206] Zhang L, Zhang Z, Wang P. NPG Asia Materials. 2012;**4**:e8

[207] Zhu H, Chen D, Li N, Xu Q, Li H, He J, Lu J. Advanced Functional Materials. 2015;**25**: 597-605

[208] Lee CH, Kang SK, Lim JA, Lim HS, Cho JH. Soft Matter. 2012;**8**:10238-10240

[209] Wu J, Jiang Y, Jiang D, He J, Cai G, Wang J. Materials Letters. 2015;**160**:384-387

[210] Li JJ, Zhou YN, Luo ZH. ACS Applied Materials and Interfaces. 2015;**7**:19643-19650

[211] Wu Y, Liu Z, Liang Y, Pei X, Zhou F, Xue Q. Langmuir. 2014;**30**:6463-6468

[212] Lv Y, Cao Y, Svec F, Tan T. Chemical Communications. 2014;**50**:13809-13812

[213] Choi I, Chi YS. Angewandte Chemie, International Edition. 2006;**45**:4894-4897

[214] Wang X, Katz E, Willner I. Electrochemical Communications. 2003;**5**:814-818

[215] Lin P, Yan F, Chan HLW. Langmuir. 2009;**25**:7465-7470

[216] Darmanin T, Guittard F. Progress in Polymer Science. 2014;**39**:656-682

[217] Darmanin T, Taffin de Givenchy E, Amigoni S, Guittard F. Advanced Materials. 2013;**25**:1378-1394

[218] Mortier C, Darmanin T, Guittard F. ChemPlusChem. 2014;**79**:1434-1439

[219] Xu L, Chen W, Mulchandani A, Yan Y. Angewandte Chemie, International Edition. 2005;**44**:6009-6012

[220] Mecerreyes D, Alvaro V, Cantero I, Bengoetxea M, Calvo PA, Grande H, Rodriguez J, Pomposo JA. Advanced Materials. 2002;**14**:749-752

[221] Chang JH, Hunter IW. Macromolecular Rapid Communications. 2011;**32**:718-723

[222] Liu M, Nie FQ, Wei Z, Song Y, Jiang L. Langmuir. 2010;**26**:3993-3997

[223] Xu L, Chen Z, Chen W, Mulchandani A, Yan Y. Macromolecular Rapid Communications. 2008;**29**:832-838

[224] Wolfs M, Darmanin T, Guittard F. Macromolecules. 2011;**44**:9286-9294

[225] Caglar A, Cengiz U, Yıldırım M, Kaya I. Applied Surface Science. 2015;**331**:262-270

[226] Xu L, Ye Q, Lu X, Lu Q. ACS Applied Materials and Interfaces. 2014;**6**:14736-14743

[227] Xu L, Lu X, Li M, Lu Q. Advanced Materials Interfaces. 2014;**1**:1400011/1-1400011/5

[228] Xu L, Chen S, Lu X, Lu Q. Macromolecular Rapid Communications. 2015;**36**:1205-1110

[229] Pernites RB, Ponnapati RR, Advincula RC. Advanced Materials. 2011;**23**:3207-3213

[230] Pernites RB, Santos CM, Maldonado M, Ponnapati RR, Rodrigues DF, Advincula RC. Chemistry of Materials. 2012;**24**:870-880

[231] Zhu Y, Hu D, Wan M, Jiang L, Wei Y. Advanced Materials. 2007;**19**:2092-2096

[232] Zhu Y, Li J, He H, Wan M, Jiang L. Macromolecular Rapid Communications. 2007; **28**:2230-2236

[233] Zhou X, Zhang Z, Xu X, Men X, Zhu X. Applied Surface Science. 2013;**276**:571-577

[234] Zhou X, Zhang Z, Men X, Yang J, Xu X, Zhu X, Xue Q. Applied Surface Science. 2011;**258**:285-289

[235] Zheng X, Guo Z, Tian D, Zhang X, Jiang L. Advanced Materials Interfaces. 2016; **3**:1600461/1-1600461/X

[236] Heng L, Guo T, Wang B, Fan LZ, Jiang L. Journal of Materials Chemistry A. 2015; **3**:23699-23706

[237] Liao J, Zhu Y, Zhou Z, Chen J, Tan G, Ning C, Mao C. Angewandte Chemie, International Edition. 2014;**53**:13068-13072

[238] Riskin M, Basnar B, Chegel VI, Katz E, Willner I, Shi F, Zhang X. Journal of the American Chemical Society. 2006;**128**:1253-1260

[239] Sinha AK, Basu M, Pradhan M, Sarkar S, Negishi Y, Pal T. Langmuir. 2011;**27**:11629-11635

[240] Wang X, Gershman Z, Kharitonov AB, Katz E, Willner I. Langmuir. 2003;**19**:5413-5420

[241] Spruijt E, Choi EY, Huck WTS. Langmuir. 2008;**24**:11253-11260

[242] Lahann J, Mitragotri S, Tran TN, Kaido H, Sundaram J, Choi IS, Hoffer S, Somorjai GA, Langer R. Science. 2003;**299**:371-374

[243] Liu Y, Mu L, Liu B, Zhang S, Yang P, Kong J. Chemical Communications. 2004:1194-1195

[244] Quinn A, Sedev R, Ralston J. Journal of Physical Chemistry B. 2003;**107**:1163-1169

[245] Im M, Kim DH, Lee JH, Yoon JB, Choi YK. Langmuir. 2010;**26**:12443-12447

[246] Krupenkin TN, Taylor JA, Schneider TM, Yang S. Langmuir. 2004;**20**:3824-3827

[247] Dhindsa MS, Smith NR, Heikenfeld J, Rack PD, Fowlkes JD, Doktycz MJ, Melechko AV, Simpson ML. Langmuir. 2006;**22**:9030-9034

[248] Zhu L, Xu J, Xiu Y, Sun Y, Hess DW, Wong CP. Journal of Physical Chemistry B. 2006;**110**:15945-15950

[249] Kakade B, Mehta R, Durge A, Kulkarni S, Pillai V. Nano Letters. 2008;**8**:2693-2696

[250] Campbell JL, Breedon M, Latham K, Kalantar-zadeh K. Langmuir. 2008;**24**:5091-5098

[251] Wu J, Xia J, Lei W, Wang BP. Applied Physics A. 2010;**99**:931-934

[252] Verplanck N, Galopin E, Camart JC, Thomy V, Coffinier Y, Boukherroub R. Nano Letters. 2007;**7**:813-817

[253] Lapierre F, Thomy V, Coffinier Y, Blossey R, Boukherroub R. Langmuir. 2009;**25**:6551-6558

[254] Brunet P, Lapierre F, Thomy V, Coffinier Y, Boukherroub R. Langmuir. 2008;**24**:11203-11208

[255] Lapierre F, Brunet P, Coffinier Y, Thomy V, Blossey R, Boukherroub R. Faraday Discussions. 2010;**146**:125-139

[256] Krupenkin TN, Taylor JA, Wang EN, Kolodner P, Hodes M, Salamon TR. Langmuir. 2007;**23**:9128-9133

[257] Manukyan G, Oh JM, Van den Ende D, Lammertink RGH, Mugele F. Physical Reviews Letters. 2011;**106**:014501/1-0145501/4

[258] Shiu JY, Chen P. Advanced Functional Materials. 2007;**17**:2680-2686

[259] Wang EN, Bucaro MA, Taylor JA, Kolodner P, Aizenberg J, Krupenkin T. Microfluidics and Nanofluidics. 2009;**7**:137-140

Chapter 8

Switchable and Reversible Superhydrophobic Surfaces: Part Two

Sabri Taleb, Thierry Darmanin and Frédéric Guittard

Additional information is available at the end of the chapter

http://dx.doi.org/10.5772/intechopen.73020

Abstract

In this book chapter, most of the methods used in the literature to prepare switchable and reversible superhydrophobic surfaces are described. Inspired by Nature, it is possible to induce the Cassie-Baxter-Wenzel transition using different external stimuli such as light, temperature, pH, ion exchange, voltage, magnetic field, mechanic stress, plasma, ultrasonication, solvent, gas or guest. Such properties are extremely important for various applications but especially for controllable oil/water separation membranes, oil-absorbing materials, and water harvesting systems.

Keywords: superhydrophobic, reversible, switchable, bioinspiration, biomimetism

1. Reversible superhydrophobic surfaces: Part two

This section provides continuation of the description of the stimuli used in the literature to induce reversible changes in surface wettability.

1.1. Ion exchange

Since 2004, the researchers have shown that the presence of charged species such as quaternary ammonium groups are sensitive to ion exchange and lead to different surface wettabilities. In 2004, Choi et al. prepared self-assembled monolayers (SAM) with imidazolium groups on smooth Au and Si/SiO_2 substrates [1–3]. They studied the effect of a series of anions as shown in **Figure 1** and they found that the surface hydrophobicity increases like this: Br^->BF_4^- >PF_6^->NO_3^->ClO_4^->TfO^->Tf_2N^-. Hence, Br^- ions led to the highest surface hydrophilicity and Tf_2N^- the highest hydrophobicity.

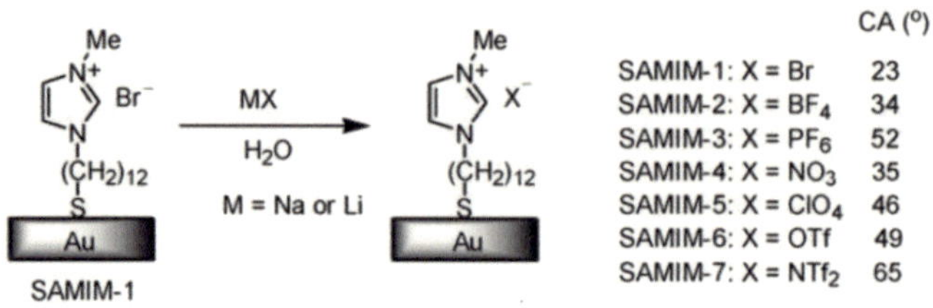

Figure 1. Grafting of monolayers on smooth gold substrates with imidazolium groups with sensitivity to ion exchange and surfaced hydrophobicity as a function of the ion-exchanged. Ref. [1], Copyright 2004. Reprinted with permission from American Chemical Society, USA.

The substituent has also an important influence on the surface wettability [3, 4]. For example, using a long substituent with 1-octyl-3-methylimidazolium ([omim]), θ_w was 68, 72, and 75° for Br^-, BF_4^- et Tf_2N^-, respectively while with 1-benzyl-3-methylimidazolium ([bmim]) θ_w did not change because the anions are absent in [bmim] aggregation. Similarly, for compounds such as 1-alkyl-3-(3-triethoxysilylpropyl)imidazolium ([C1tespim]) (**Figure 1**), θ_w was 24, 30, and 42° for Cl^-, BF_4^- et PF_6^-, respectively while with ([C4tespim]) θ_w did not change. Moreover, the cation nature has also an influence on the surface hydrophobicity [3].

In order to elaborate reversible superhydrophobic properties by ion exchange, gold micro and nanostructured substrates were performed by electroless etching process by immersing silicon substrates in aqueous solution of $HAuCl_4$ and HF (**Figure 2**). The surface was then modified by SAM using a thiol terminated by a quaternary ammonium. Then, the surface wettability could be reversely changed from superhydrophilic to superhydrophobic after exchanging Cl^- ions by perfluorooctanoate ($C_7F_{15}COO^-$ or PFO^-) ions [4].

Moreover, polymers with charged species such as polyelectrolytes were also used to change the surface wettability [5–15]. For example, [PVBIm][PF_6] ([1-(4-vinylbenzyle)-3-butylimidazolium hexafluorophosphate]) brushes were grafted on a silicon wafer by atom transfer radical polymerization (ATRP). The surface properties could be changed from hydrophobic (θ_w = 95°) to hydrophilic (θ_w = 41°) after exchanging PF_6^- ions by Cl^- ions. The wettability of polyelectrolyte

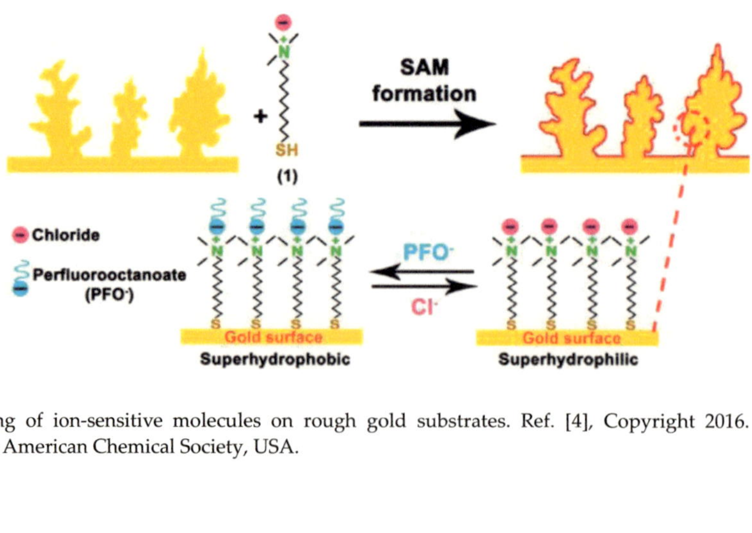

Figure 2. Grafting of ion-sensitive molecules on rough gold substrates. Ref. [4], Copyright 2016. Reprinted with permission from American Chemical Society, USA.

brushes could be modified with appropriate counter-ions [12–15] using poly(2-methacryl poly oxyethyl trimethylammonium chloride) (PMETAC) and poly(2-dimethylaminoethyl methacrylate chloride) (PDMAEMAC).

Superhydrophobic properties could be reached by grafting PMETAC on gold micro and nanostructured substrates by ATRP [16]. Then, reversible and switchable properties from superhydrophobic to superhydrophilic were obtained after exchanging Tf_2N^- ions by SCN^- ions. PMETAC were also grafted onto the surface of multiwalled carbon nanotubes [17]. Their surface properties could be reversely changed from superhydrophobic/highly oleophobic to superhydrophilic/superoleophobic after exchanging PFO^- ions by SCN^- ions. PMETAC was also grafted on cotton fabrics leading to similar properties [18]. Zhang et al. fabricated first silicone nanofilaments and modified them by P(METAC-*co*-trifluoroethyl methacrylate) to the obtained reversible surface [19].

Cho et al. developed a multifunctional polyelectrolyte membranes by electrospinning of P(METAC-*co*-[trimethoxysilyl]propylmethacrylate) (PMETAC-*co*-TSPM) [20]. Here, the presence of TSPM (sol-gel precursor) was used not only to form a polymer network *via* intramolecular interactions but also to anchor substrates (**Figure 3**). The membranes could reversely change from superhydrophobic/highly oleophobic to superhydrophilic/superoleophobic after exchanging Cl^- ions by heptadecafluorooctanesulfonic acid ($C_8F_{17}SO_3^-$ or HPS^-) ions. Moreover, the membranes were also highly efficient filter medium for removing multiple contaminants such as SO_2 form waster gas streams. Another strategy was to deposit polyelectrolyte multilayers poly(diallyldimethylammonium chloride (PDDA) and poly(sodium 4-styrenesulfonate) (PSS) on gold micro and nanostructured substrates [21]. The authors studied the influence of the exchanged ions and the highest properties were obtained by exchanging Cl^- ($\theta_w < 5°$) ions by PFO^- ($\theta_w = 164°$). The authors also deposited polyelectrolyte multilayers on micro and nanostructured aluminum substrates obtained by etching in HCl and immersion in boiling water [22, 23]. Using PFO^- ions, the substrates were superhydrophobic and superoleophobic. When the substrates were immersed in seawater, the PFO^- ions were exchanged by hydrophilic Cl^- or SO_4^{2-} making the substrates underwater superoleophobic.

1.2. Magnetic field

Environment protection against oil leakage during oil tankers sinking is a major global problem. Finding new materials to separate oil/water mixtures is hence extremely important [24–26]. Athanassiou et al. reported the formation of a novel composite material based on polyurethane (PU) foams functionalized with colloidal superparamagnetic iron oxide (spinel-cubic γ-Fe_2O_3/Fe_3O_4) nanoparticles and submicrometer PTFE particles [27]. The resulting foams could efficiently separate oil from water. The combination of the functionalization of the PTFE-treated foam surfaces with colloidal iron oxide nanoparticles significantly increased the speed of oil absorption. The foams were also magnetically responsive because they could be magnetically actuated. Durable and magnetic PU sponges were also reported by CVD of tetraethoxysilane (TEOS) to bind Fe_3O_4 nanoparticles [28]. The sponges exhibited fast magnetic responsivity with a saturation magnetization of 22.73 emu/g and can be easily manipulated with a magnet. The sponges were also superhydrophobic and superoleophilic, quickly absorbed floating oils on the water surface and also displayed high mechanical properties.

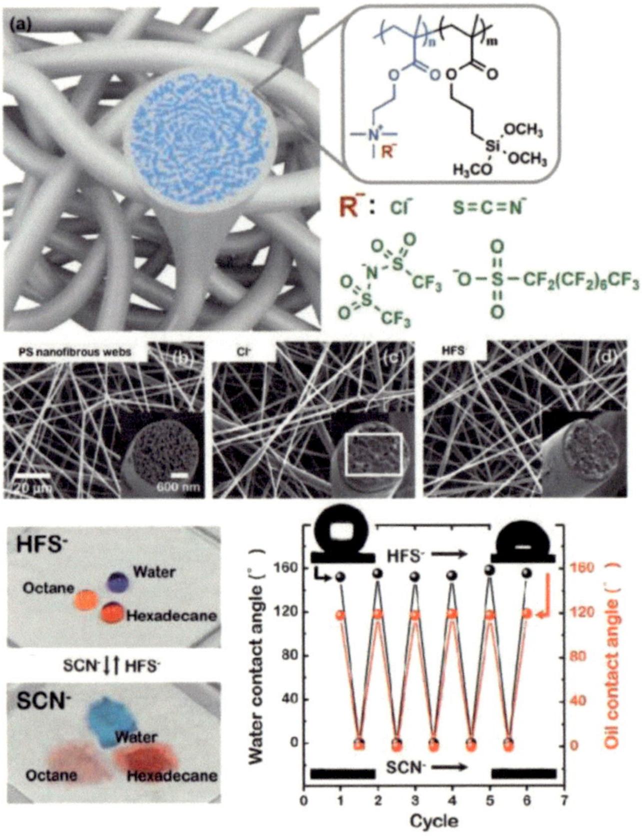

Figure 3. Membranes sensitivity to ion exchange prepared by electrospinning of PMETAC-co-TSPM. The resulting membranes could switch from superhydrophobic/highly oleophobic to superhydrophilic/superoleophobic by changing the counter-ions. Ref. [20], copyright 2012. Reprinted with permission from Royal Society of Chemistry, United Kingdom.

Other materials were also used in the literature [29–35]. Inspired by marine mussel adhesive, Jiang et al. used dopamine to link Fe_3O_4 nanoparticles on electrospun PVDF [29]. After fluorination, the materials displayed oil adsorption properties and could move towards a magnet. Using magnetically responsive mesh substrates, micro-robots were fabricated (**Figure 4**) [30]. The meshes could float and move on air/water and oil/water interfaces and could be guided by a magnetic field.

Zhang et al. reported superamphiphobic elastic and magnetic silicone sponges with excellent thermal stability [31]. Their sponges were prepared by hydrolytic condensation of methyltrimethoxysilane, dimethoxydimethylsilane in the presence of Fe_3O_4@SiO_2 nanoparticles and finally fluorinated. Superhydrophobic and magnetic quartz fibers were also reported by loading in cobalt and modification with PDMS [32].

Another potential application of magnetically responsive materials is the control of liquid moving using a magnet [36]. Randomly oriented hierarchical arrays with control geometries (diameter, height, and density) could be prepared by the mouldless self-assembly of solutions

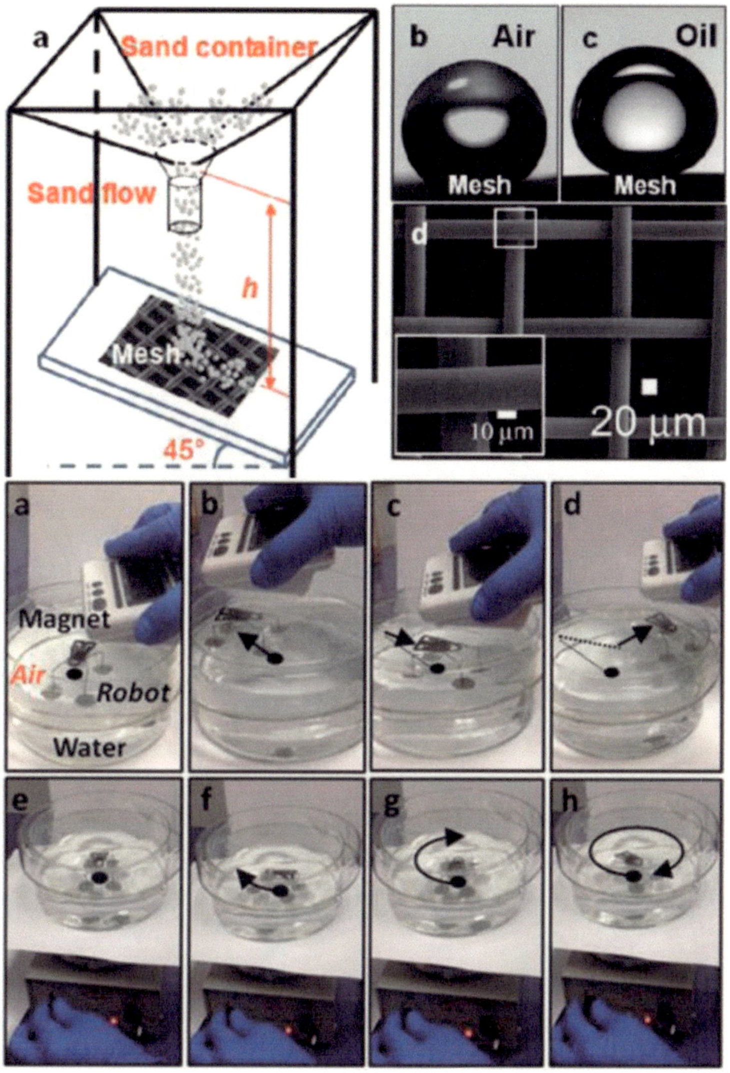

Figure 4. Fabrication of micro-robots using magnetically responsive mesh substrates and Fe_3O_4 nanoparticles. Ref. [30], Copyright 2015. Reprinted with permission from Royal Society of Chemistry, United Kingdom.

comprising procured polymers and magnetic particles under a magnetic field. With their actuating and superhydrophobic properties, these flexible films enabled active, fast, precise, and reversible manipulation of droplets with the use of a magnet.

Moreover, using superparamagnetic droplets on a magnetic superhydrophobic film, it was also shown to switch from superhydrophobic (low adhesion) to parahydrophobic (high adhesion) properties after magnetization/demagnetization [37]. It is also possible to control the speed, the shape, and the self-assembly of magnetic droplets on the superhydrophobic surface by modulating the magnetic field (**Figure 5**) [38, 39].

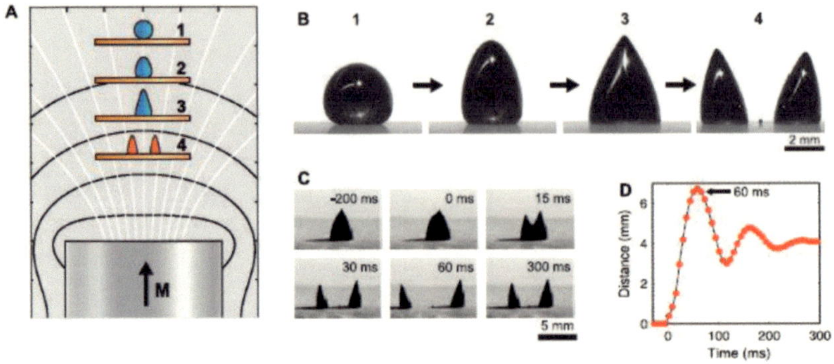

Figure 5. Modification of the speed, the shape and the self-assembly of magnetic droplets on the superhydrophobic surface by modulating the magnetic field. Ref. [38], Copyright 2013. Reprinted with permission from The American Association for the Advancement of Science, United Kingdom.

1.3. Mechanical stress

Most of the time, reversible switchable wettability is governed by the change in the surface chemistry (surface energy). However, the use of mechanical strains is a very interesting way to control the surface wettability by modifying the surface roughness. In 2004, Zhang et al. showed that the hydrophobicity of PTFE can reversely change from 108 to 165° as the material is extended to 190% [40]. This was attributed to an increase in the distance between the fibrous PTFE crystals. They also described a novel method to reversibly change the wettability (from superhydrophilic to superhydrophobic) of a polyamide film with a triangular net-like structure upon biaxial extension and unloading [41]. The average side-length of the triangular structures was around 200 μm before extension and the surface was superhydrophobic, and 450 μm and superhydrophilic after extension. The phenomena could be repeated around 20 times because the film had a good elasticity.

Using a flexible PDMS with micropillar arrays, it was reported the feasibility to drastic change the surface wettability by simple modification of the substrate curvature (**Figure 6**) [42, 43]. When the substrate was not incurved it was parahydrophobic (high water adhesion) while it became superhydrophobic after curvature become the curvature could induce air injection into the pillar arrays. This easy and reversible process could be used in microfluidic devices [42–45].

To obtain micro and nanostructures on PDMS, Singh et al. deposited Ag nanorods arrays using oblique angle deposition on prestretched PDMS (**Figure 7**) [46]. The substrates displayed both microbuckles/wrinkles and nanorods. Superhydrophobic properties with θ_w = 154.8° under 30% prestretching, which is due to optimal amplitude and periodicity of the wrinkles. The substrates also displayed anisotropic wetting and water droplets could move only along the direction parallel to the wrinkles. Reversible contact angles from 154.8 to 126.2° were also reported by simple stretching/relaxation cycles because the stretching changes the dimensions of the microstructures. Yang et al. also reported the properties of PDMS elastomers with microscale ripples and SiO_2 nanoparticles, allowing to reach anisotropic superhydrophobic properties [47]. The surface properties were dependent on the ripple amplitude and periodicity and also on the surface chemistry. Here, the sliding angle could also reversibly be tuned with external strains and with fast response.

http://dx.doi.org/10.5772/intechopen.73020

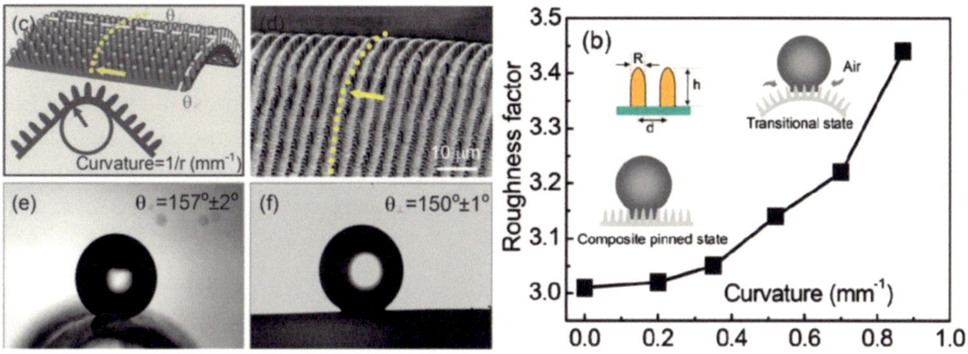

Figure 6. Change in the water adhesion by inducing flexion on a flexible micro-patterned substrate. Ref. [43], Copyright 2011. Reprinted with permission from AIP Publishing LLC, USA.

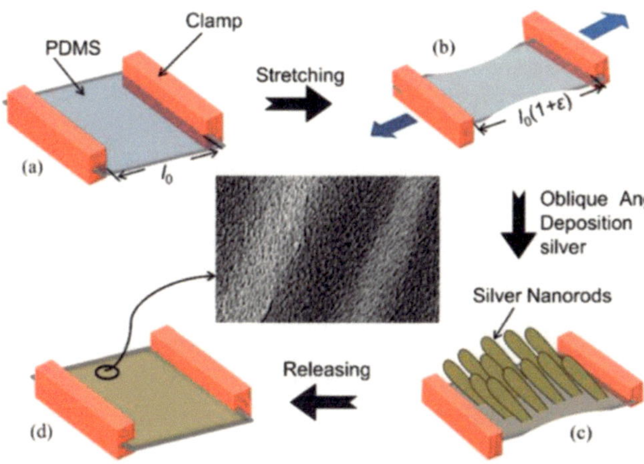

Figure 7. Preparation of microwrinkles of PDMS by pre-stretching following by oblique angle deposition of Ag nanorod. Ref. [46], Copyright 2015. Reprinted with permission from American Chemical Society, USA.

Self-healing superhydrophobic textiles with mechanical responsivity were also reported [48]. To induce this property, polydopamine nanocapsules with trapped hydrophobic agents were coated on the textiles. The nanocapsules could be released using different mechanical stresses, such as stretching, compression, friction, and even mechanical washing, and lead to self-healing properties.

1.4. Plasma

In a plasma chamber, highly ionized species are created by applying an electric field between two electrodes. When the plasma interacts with a substrate, different effects can be produced such as the surface cleaning, the formation of chemical groups, and/or the formation of surface structures. These effects are highly dependent on the plasma parameters such as the used gas, the pressure or the power and also on the substrate nature. For example, if a hydrophobic monolayer is used to prepare a superhydrophobic surface, the plasma treatment can remove the monolayer and leads to superhydrophobic properties [49–52].

However, to obtain reversible properties, it is often necessary to have again the hydrophobic monolayer and/or to storage in the dark.

Otherwise, following the used gas, the plasma treatment can also change the surface chemistry. For example, meshes substrates were coated by CVD with the nanocrystalline diamond film [53]. After H_2 plasma, the surface diamond termination changed with hydrogen atom leading to superhydrophobic properties. Moreover, the surface properties were reversible by annealing in air at 500°C.

1.5. Ultrasound

Very recently, full reversibility between the Cassie-Baxter and Wenzel states were reported through acoustic pressure [54]. Ultrasonication is used both for the nucleation of bubbles directly on superhydrophobic surfaces. Oppositely, the collapse of an entrapped air film was promoted to reversibly manipulate the material surface properties and the interaction with the environment.

1.6. Guest

It is known that specific interactions between "guest" and "host" molecules can be extremely strong. This is the case, for example, between crown ethers and ions. Li et al. used this strategy to develop superhydrophobic surfaces with specific sensitivity [55]. They grafted by click chemistry calix[4]azacrown (C4AC) on micro/nanostructured silicon substrates. Different organic ion pairs were selected (**Figure 8**): 1-butyl-3-methylimidazolium (C_4mim) with different counter ions (Cl^-, Br^- and PF_6^-). Reversible surfaces from superhydrophobic to superhydrophilic were observed but only in the presence of [C_4mim]Cl because [C_4mim]Cl interacts with C4AC cavities and cone resulting in 1,3-alternate conversion. Calix[4]arene lipoic acid (C4LA) was also grafted on the gold substrate [56]. The substrate had specific interaction with guest molecules, resulting in a high decrease of surface hydrophobicity. The interaction was specific with methomyl (a carbamate pesticide) but not with four other tested carbamate pesticides. With the aim to remove metal ions from the environment, responsive mesh was prepared by coating with poly(acrylic acid) hydrogel [57]. The resulting mesh was superhydrophilic and underwater superoleophobic. The mesh could complex Hg^+ ions by complexation with the COO^- groups of poly(acrylic acid) leading to an increase in water contact angle and a decrease in underwater oil contact angle.

Metal-organic frameworks (MOFs), also known as porous coordination polymers, were also used in the literature. In order to prepare hydrophobic MOFs, Planas et al. used an *ortho*-carborane functionalized with pyridylmethyl alcohol groups at the C-positions as a hydrophobic linker to Zn-1,4-benzenedicarboxylate [58]. Moreover, the substrate could change from highly hydrophobic to superhydrophilic by immersion in NaOH/DMF. In order to obtain fluorescent and hydrophobic MOFS, pyrene was incorporated in the structure [59]. The resulting materials displayed super-absorbency and could remove oils from oil/water mixture. They could also C_{60} as guest offering great promise for application in sensors.

In order to develop biosensors with switchable wettability, different strategies were used in order to bind biological molecules. For that, a tricomponent copolymer containing

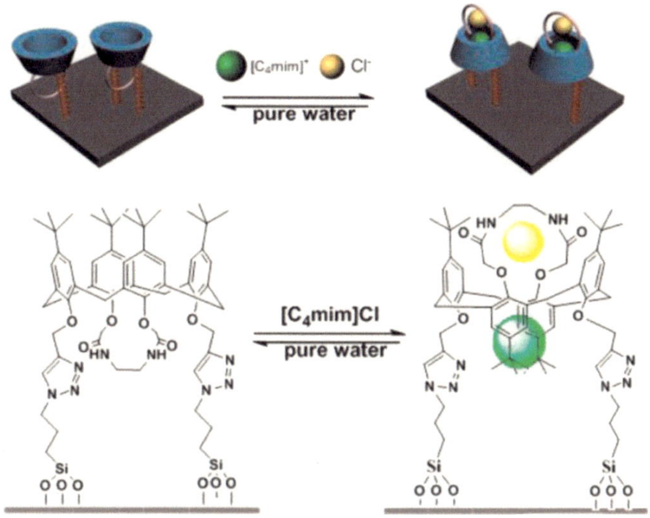

Figure 8. Preparation of guest-responsive surface using calix[4]azacrown derivatives. Ref. [55], Copyright 2012. Reprinted with permission from American Chemical Society, USA.

phenylthiourea and phenylboronic acid was designed [60]. As a strong hydrogen-bonding donor, phenylthiourea was used to combine with the phosphate units and phenylboronic acid to combine with the pentose rings. The copolymer was grafted on structured silicon substrates. The substrates could switch from superhydrophobic to superhydrophilic after immersion in adenosine diphosphate (ADP) aqueous solution. Using copolymers with phenylboronic acid units, biosensors that can bind sugars such as glucose were also reported in the literature [61].

1.7. Solvent and gas

When structured polymer materials are immersed into a solvent such as water, the interactions between the polymer chains and in contact with the solvent can highly varied leading to possible changes in surface morphology and wettability. Mixed polymer brushes with hydrophobic and hydrophilic blocks were used and fixed to a substrate. After exposure to different solvents, the organization of these chains can be highly affected as shown in **Figure 9** [62, 63]. As a consequence, the surface energy and as a consequence θ_w vary [64, 65].

To verify this hypothesis, molecules in Y-shape composed of hydrophobic polystyrene PS and hydrophilic poly(acrylic acid) (PAA) were grafted on a substrate [66, 67]. When the substrate was immersed in toluene, a good solvent for PS, the layer at the extreme surface was mainly composed of PS brushes and reversely the orientation of the polymers chains could highly vary as a function of the affinity with the solvent. PAA-block-PS was also grafted on multiwall carbon nanotubes. The surface could reversely switch from superhydrophobic to parahydrophobic by immersion in water and heating [68].

In order to reach superhydrophobic properties, Minko et al. grafted carboxyl-terminated poly(styrene-*co*-2,3,4,5,6-pentafluorostyrene) (PSF-COOH) and carboxyl-terminated poly(2-vinylpyridine) (PVP-COOH) on flat and rough (with needle-like structures) PTFE substrates functionalized with hydroxyl and amino groups (**Figure 10**) [69, 70]. After exposure to toluene,

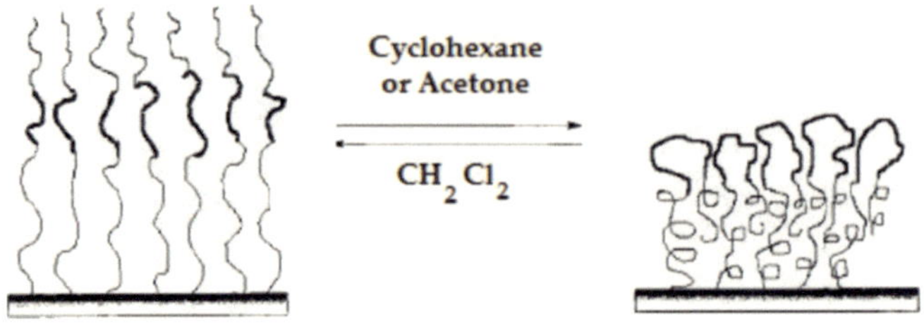

Figure 9. Changing in the organization of mixed polymer brushes with hydrophobic and hydrophilic blocks after exposure to different solvents. Ref. [63], Copyright 2002. Reprinted with permission from American Chemical Society, USA.

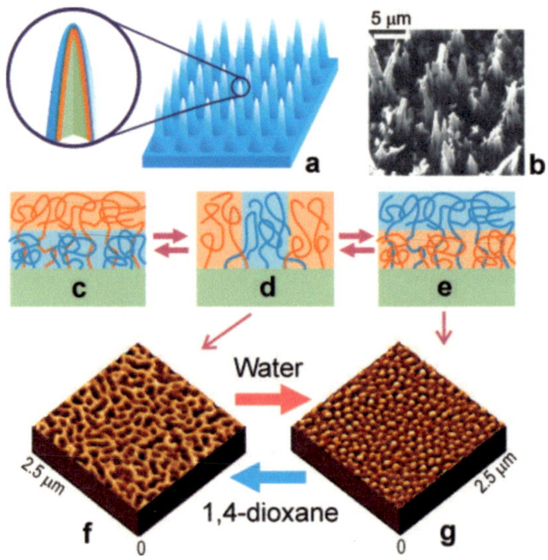

Figure 10. Change in the surface topography and organization of needle-like PTFE nanostructures grafted with PSF-COOH and PVP-COOH after exposure to different solvents. Ref. [70], Copyright 2003. Reprinted with permission from American Chemical Society, USA.

the top layer was mainly composed of hydrophobic PSF while after exposure to water the surface topography changed: PSF formed round domains inside the hydrophilic PVP matrix. As a consequence, on flat substrates, θ_w varies from 118 to 25° while on rough substrates θ_w varies from 160 to 0°.

Ji et al. developed an asymmetric free-standing film layer-by-layer (LbL) assembly using polyethyleneimine (PEI) and PAA [71]. After coating with Teflon on one side, the free-standing film was superhydrophobic on one side and hydrophilic on the other side. As a function of the humidity, the free-standing film could be in a control manner bended and unbended (**Figure 11**). In a similar manner, Sun et al. developed films that could reversely induce wrinkles in the presence of humidity by depositing hydrophobic SiO_2 nanoparticles on multilayer assembly of poly(allylamine hydrochloride) (PAH) and PAA [72]. Aizenberg et al. also reported a very innovative strategy by embedding nanoarrays in a hydrogel [73]. When the material was exposed to water, the orientation of the nanostructures changes leading to different surface hydrophobicity.

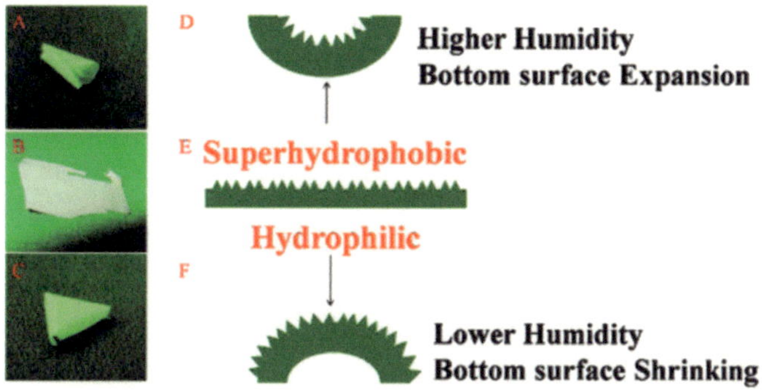

Figure 11. Control in the bending of free-standing films prepared by LbL of PEI and PAA as a function of humidity. Ref. [71], Copyright 2010. Reprinted with permission from American Chemical Society, USA.

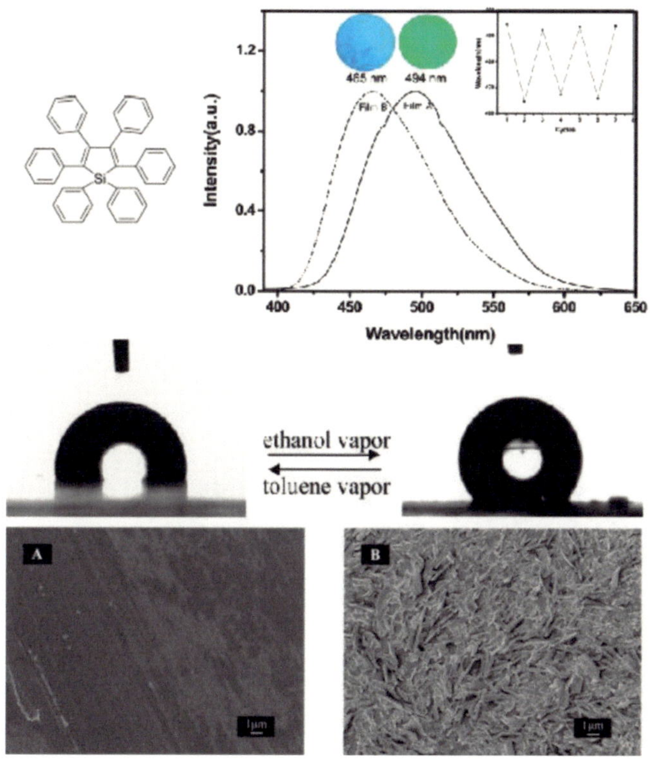

Figure 12. Reversible control in the surface structuration, hydrophobicity, and luminescence properties of 1,2,3,4,5-hexaphenylsilole films after exposure to ethanol vapor and toluene vapor, respectively. Ref. [74], Copyright 2008. Reprinted with permission from American Chemical Society, USA.

Tang et al. reported that 1,2,3,4,5-hexaphenylsilole is a unique solvent-sensitive material with switchable luminescence properties (**Figure 12**) [74]. When this material is spin-coated on a substrate, the resulting material is smooth, slightly hydrophobic ($\theta_w = 97.0°$) and displayed a green light luminescence. After exposure to ethanol vapor, the substrate became nanostructured, highly hydrophobic (θ_w = 136.3°) and displayed a blue light luminescence. Moreover, the surface properties could be reversely switched using toluene vapor.

Inorganic materials can also be used to obtain solvent-sensitive but, here, it is often possible when interactions of the substrates with the solvent induce changes in the surface chemistry [75–77]. This is the case of titanate nanostructures in water. The authors reported a change in the surface hydrophobicity due to physically adsorbed water molecules [75]. Moreover, the surface was reversible by simple heating. Otherwise, the immersion of inorganic materials can also lead to the removal of the hydrophobic treatment and as a consequence highly decreases the surface hydrophobicity [78, 79].

Different materials sensitive to gases were also reported in the literature [80–86]. 19-25 Jiang et al. developed superhydrophobic indium hydroxide ($InOH)_3$) with microcubes and nanorods using a hydrothermal process in the presence of $InCl_3$ and urea (**Figure 13**) [80]. The surface could switch from superhydrophobic to superhydrophilic in the presence of ammonia ($NH_3{\cdot}H_2O$). Indeed, $In(OH)_3$ being acidic, the ammonia molecules would anchor to the surface and form an ammonia layer on the surface of $In(OH)_3$. Moreover, the bonds created between $In(OH)_3$ and $NH_3.H_2O$ being weak, they can be easily broken by heating leading again to superhydrophobic properties. $In(OH)_3$-PDMS sponges with NH_3 sensitivity were also prepared in the presence of polydopamine [81]. In a similar manner, CO_2 is an acid gas; it can react at the surface of a material if amine groups are present. This strategy was used by Yuan et al. [83]. They electrospun PMMA-*co*-poly(*N*,*N*-dimethylaminoethyl methacrylate), a copolymer with amine groups. The resulting materials could switch from highly hydrophobic and underwater oleophobic to highly hydrophilic and underwater oleophilic in the presence of CO_2. Moreover,

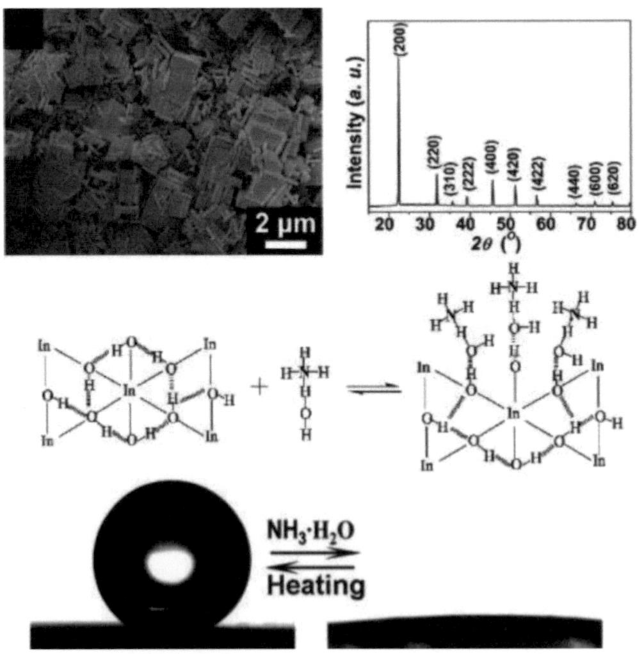

Figure 13. Influence of $NH_3{\cdot}H_2O$ on the surface hydrophobicity of $In(OH)_3$ with microcubes and nanorods. Ref. [80], Copyright 2008. Reprinted with permission from American Chemical Society, USA.

the properties were reversible in the presence of N_2. A very interesting work was reported by Wang et al. using the allochroic material (a material that can changes color) crystal violet lactone (CVL) [84]. To obtain superhydrophobic properties, palygorskite@polysiloxane was modified with CVL. The resulting materials could change from blue (CVL^+: the carboxylate group of CVL) to discolored (CVL) in the presence of different gas vapor such as acetone.

A palladium-based superhydrophobic substrate was reported by Pd coating on vertically aligned Si nanowires [85]. The resulting substrates could reversely switch from superhydrophobic to parahydrophobic (high adhesion) properties in the presence of H_2 or air, respectively. Here, the changes are due to a change in the surface energy due to the formation of β-phase Pd hydride (PdH_x). Moreover, the substrates could potentiate the therapeutic efficiency of 3D stem cell spheroids. ZnO nanowires could also be reversely switched from superhydrophobic to superhydrophilic in the presence of O_2 and H_2, respectively, but at high temperature (300°C) [86]. Using a model based on density functional theory, the authors showed that oxygen-related defects are responsible for the wettability switching.

1.8. Chemical reactions

Different grafting strategies can also be envisaged to prepare the surface with reversible wettability [87–89]. For example, nanofibers of poly(3,4-ethylenedioxythiophene) (PEDOT) functionalized with azido groups (N_3) were prepared by electropolymerization [87]. Then, dithiolane groups were introduced by reaction with lipoic acid also called thioctic acid. Then, various thiols were introduced to modify the surface properties. Both the surface morphology and the surface hydrophobicity were affected by the post-treatment with the used thiol. Interestingly, the use of fluorinated thiols highly changed the surface morphology and porosity leading to superhydrophobic properties and highly oleophobic properties. Moreover, the surface hydrophobicity and oleophobicity were reversible by reaction with dithiothreitol (DTT) to form the dithiolane groups again (**Figure 14**).

The boronic ester chemistry was also used to reversely change the surface properties [88]. This time, nanostructured PEDOT films functionalized with protected 1,2-diol were prepared by electropolymerization. After deprotection, the surface could easily react with different boronic acids containing different aromatic groups as shown in **Figure 15**. Similarly, both the surface morphology and the surface hydrophobicity were affected by the use of boronic acid post-treatment. The highest properties were obtained with the pyrene group for which the surface was parahydrophobic (extremely high water adhesion) with $\theta_w = 135°$.

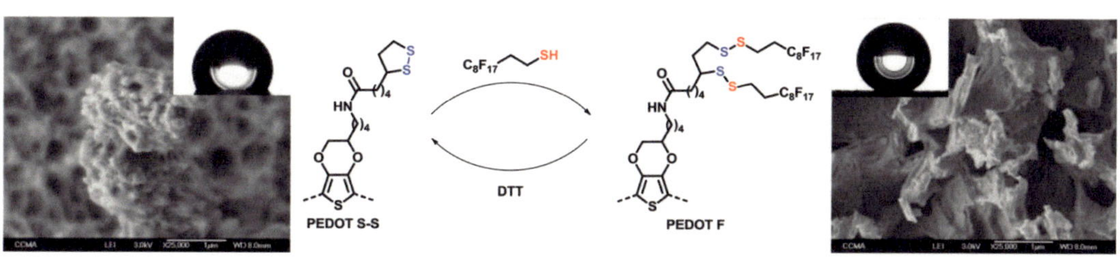

Figure 14. Reversible wetting properties by reaction of hydrophobic thiols on dithiolane and DTT [87].

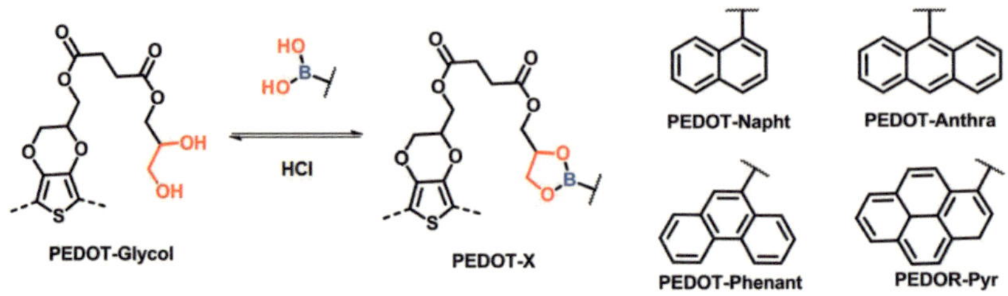

Figure 15. Reversible wetting properties by reaction of hydrophobic boronic acids on 1,2-diols and HCl [88].

1.9. Dual sensitivity

Temperature and pH: Switchable surfaces by temperature and pH were prepared using thermosensitive polymers functionalized by pH-sensitive groups such as carboxylic acids (COOH) or amines. For example, a copolymer of poly(*N*-isopropylacrylamide) (PNIPAAm: sensitive to temperature) and polyacrylic acid (PAA: sensitive to pH) was grafted on micro and nanostructured silicon substrates (**Figure 16**) [90, 91]. The resulting surface could switch from superhydrophobic (low adhesion) at high temperature (45°C) and/or low pH (2) to parahydrophobic (high adhesion) at low temperature (20°C) and/or high pH (11).

Different polymers with amino or pyridinium groups were also used to induce pH sensitivity [92–96]. Hybrid responsive nanoparticles were prepared by grafting on a SiO_2 core mixed block copolymers of PS and poly(4-vinylpyridine) (P4VP) [92, 93]. PS is a thermosensitive polymer

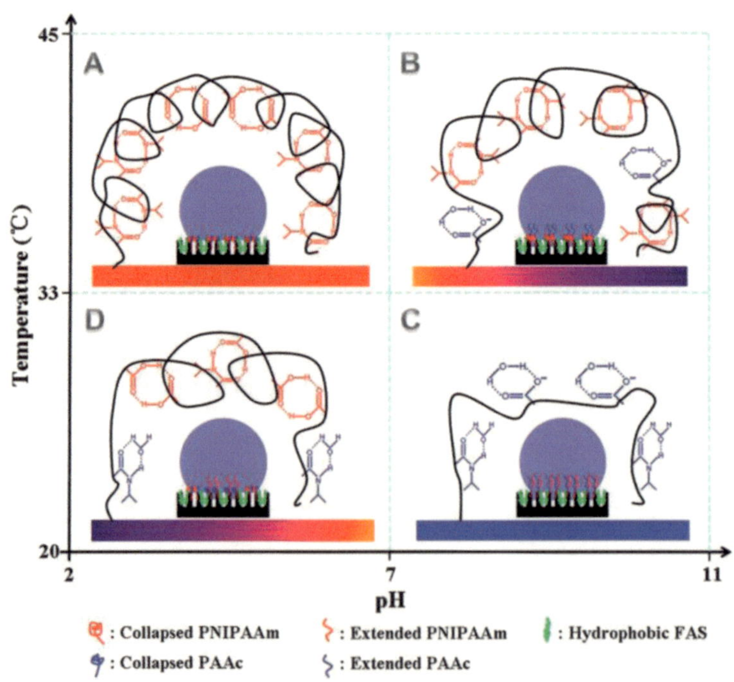

Figure 16. Temperature and pH-switchable surfaces using PNIPAAm and PAA copolymers. Ref. [90], Copyright 2012. Reprinted with permission from Royal Society of Chemistry, United Kingdom.

with a Tg of 100°C while P4VP is sensitive to pH. The surface was superhydrophobic at high pH (6) and at a temperature (> 100°C) while θ_w decreased with the temperature and pH. The authors also observed that the surface roughness changed with the temperature and pH. Wang et al. modified stainless steel meshes with a hydrogel copolymer of 2-(dimethylamino)ethyl methacrylate and methacrylic acid (two monomers sensitive to pH) [95]. Using oil/water mixtures, the meshes could let water pass through with a separation efficiency of 98.35% but only at both high temperature (55°C) and low pH (7), or both low temperature (25°C) and high pH (13). Poly-L-lysine, as both pH and the thermosensitive peptide, was also tested on a micro and nanostructured silicon substrate [96]. The surface was superhydrophobic at both high temperature (60°C) and high pH (11.5), and became superhydrophilic as the temperature and/or the pH decrease.

Solvent and pH: To prepare polymer particles responsive to solvent and pH, copolymers were prepared using a hydrophilic moiety (PAA) and hydrophobic ones (poly(2,3,4,5,6-pentafluorostyrene) [97]. The polymer films produced by annealing in the air led to superhydrophobic properties while by annealing in water led to highly hydrophilic properties (**Figure 17**). This was due to the reorientation of the PAA groups in water. Moreover, due to the presence of COOH groups, the pH could also modify the surface charge between negative and neutral, which can also modify the surface hydrophobicity.

Voltage and pH: Switchable surfaces by voltage and pH were prepared using conducting polymers for their sensitivity to voltage. First, polyaniline was used for its sensitivity also to pH [98, 99]. To form superhydrophobic micro and nanostructured polyaniline with urchin-like and core-shell structures, polystyrene microspheres were used as seed (hard template) for the growth of polyaniline nanofibers [98]. The surface could switch from superhydrophobic to superhydrophilic depending on the voltage and the pH. Similar properties were also reported on polyaniline-polyacrylonitrile coaxial nanofibers prepared by electrospinning [99].

Switchable surface from superhydrophobic properties to highly hydrophilic were obtained by electro-copolymerization of PEDOT monomers with both pH-sensitive groups (COOH)

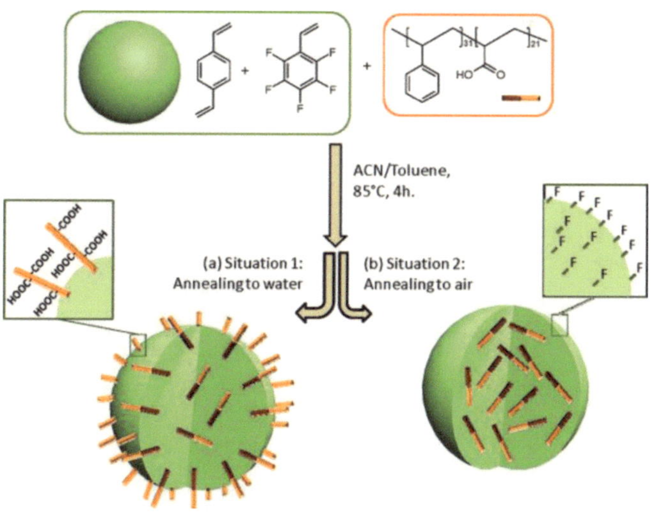

Figure 17. Solvent and pH-switchable surfaces using poly(2,3,4,5,6-pentafluorostyrene) and PAA copolymers. Ref. [97], Copyright 2010. Reprinted with permission from American Chemical Society, USA.

and fluorinated chains [100]. The authors studied the influence of the percentage of each monomer, the doping state and also the pH on both the surface hydrophobicity (**Figure 18**). The surface morphology changed with the percentage of each monomer. The highest wettability changes were observed for a mol% of EDOT-COOH between 12.5 and 25%.

Voltage and Ion Exchange: Switchable surfaces by voltage and ion exchange were prepared using conducting polymers for their sensitivity to voltage while the sensitivity to ion exchange could be obtained by introducing functional groups such as ammonium, imidazolium or sulfonate groups. For example, multiresponsive surfaces were obtained by grafting an imidazolium substituent on PEDOT polymers [101, 102]. Smooth polymer films were prepared by spin-coating and observed sensitivity to ion exchange, oxidative doping, temperature, and pH. Their surface hydrophobicity could be modified from 40 to 70–72° by exchanging the counter-anion of the imidazolium moiety with fluorinated bis(trifluoromethane)sulfonamide or nonafluoro-1-butanesulfonate anions. The surface properties could be also enhanced from 24 to 107° by depositing the polymer on ZnO nanowire arrays. The surface properties of PEDOT:PSS were also studied by the authors [103].

In order to reach superhydrophobic properties, PEDOT copolymers with both ion exchange functional groups and fluorinated chains were prepared by electro-copolymerization (**Figure 19**) [104, 106]. The authors studied the influence of the percentage of each monomer, the doping state and also the counter-ions of ion exchange functional groups on both the surface hydrophobicity (**Figure 19**) [104]. Surprisingly, using 25 mol% of EDOT-Py⁺, the surface could switch from superhydrophobic to hydrophilic by reduction (dedoping using a different voltage) and again

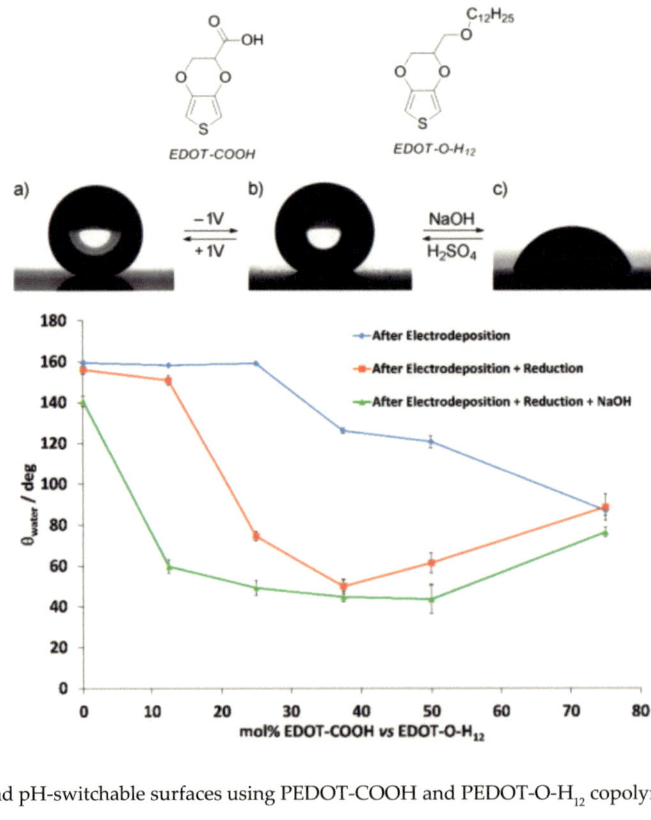

Figure 18. Voltage and pH-switchable surfaces using PEDOT-COOH and PEDOT-O-H_{12} copolymers [101].

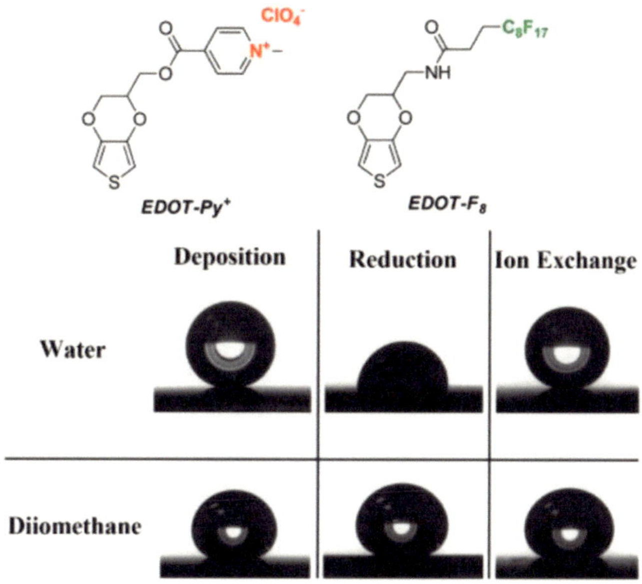

Figure 19. Voltage and ion exchange-switchable surfaces using PEDOT-Py+ and PEDOT-F_8 copolymers [104].

superhydrophobic properties by ions exchange with hydrophobic bis(trifluoromethanesulfonyl) imide (Tf_2N^-) ions while the superoleophobic properties remained unchanged. Hence, it was possible to obtain both superoleophobic and hydrophilic properties, which is extremely rare in the literature [105]. Moreover, superoleophobic properties were also prepared with poly(3,4-ethylenedioxypyrrole) PEDOP copolymers with ion exchange functional groups and fluorinated chains [106].

Light and ion exchange: Switchable surfaces by light and ion exchange were reported by SAM of an imidazolium moiety (sensitive to ion exchange) terminated with a fluorinated chain on nanostructured ZnO (sensitive to light) films [107]. The authors studied the influence of ZnO morphology, the counter-ions (I^-, BF_4^-, PF_6^-, Tf_2N^-) of imidazolium groups and the light on the surface hydrophobicity. Superhydrophobic properties were obtained with ZnO nanoparticles and hydrophobic PF_6^- or Tf_2N^- ions. Moreover, the surface could reversely switch from superhydrophobic to hydrophilic by UV irradiation and dark storage.

Mechanic stress and magnetic field: Liu et al. developed flexible conical arrays coated with magnetic nanoparticles for fog harvesting systems [108]. Under an external magnetic field, static fog water could be spontaneously and continuously captured and directionally transported from the tip to the base of the spine through periodic vibration of the flexible conical spines driven by the magnetic field and the Laplace pressure difference arising from the conical shape of the flexible spines (**Figure 20**). Magnetically sensitive superomniphobic surfaces were also reported by fabricating flexible micronail caps [109]. The micronail caps could reversely bend using an external magnetic field, which changed the surface properties from superomniphobic to superomniphilic.

Multiresponsivity: Switchable surfaces with responsivity to both light, heat, and pH was prepared by modifying TiO_2 (sensitive to light) nanoparticles with a copolymer of poly(*N*-isopropylacrylamide) (PNIPAAm: sensitive to temperature) and polyacrylic acid (PAA: sensitive to pH) [110].

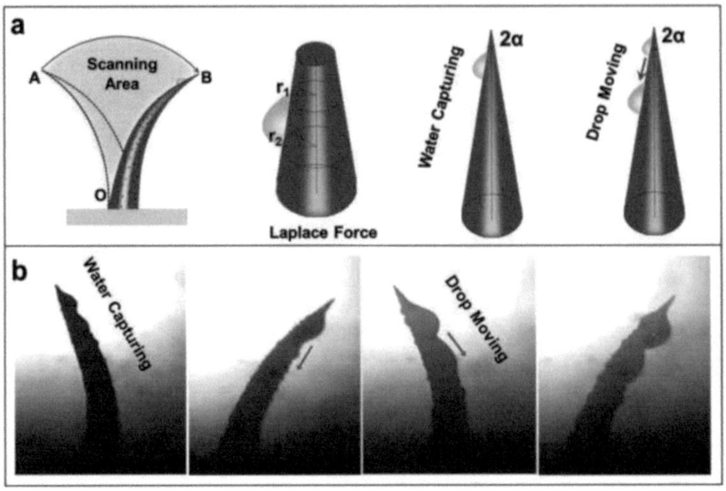

Figure 20. Switchable surfaces with mechanic stress and magnetic field by creating flexible magnetic conical arrays [108].

The resulting polymer surfaces displayed reversible wettability from superhydrophobic to superhydrophilic by UV and heat treatment at 150°C or immersion in solution of pH 12 and 2. Multiresponsive surfaces to heat, pH, and sugars was also reported by using a copolymer of PNIPAAm (sensitive to temperature) and poly(acrylamidophenylboronic acid (sensitive to both sugars and pH) [111]. The surface could switch from superhydrophobic to superhydrophilic by cooling at T = 20°C, exposure to glucose or immersion at high pH (10.1).

2. Conclusion

In this book chapter, most of the articles dedicated to switchable and reversible superhydrophobic surfaces were reviewed. If superhydrophobic properties are highly present in Nature, the preparation of reversible superhydrophobic properties has become one of the most studied domains. Indeed, if robust superhydrophobic surfaces can be obtained if the surface structures are able to stabilize the Cassie-Baxter state, it is possible to induce the Cassie-Baxter-Wenzel transition. In the literature, various techniques were developed to control the surface wettability using extern stimuli such as light, temperature, pH, ion exchange, voltage, magnetic field, mechanic stress, plasma, ultrasonication, solvent, gas or guest. Such properties are extremely important for various applications but especially for controllable oil/water separation membranes, oil-absorbing materials, and water harvesting systems.

Author details

Sabri Taleb, Thierry Darmanin* and Frédéric Guittard

*Address all correspondence to: thierry.darmanin@unice.fr

NICE Lab, IMREDD, Université Côte d'Azur, Nice, France

References

[1] Lee BS, Chi YS, Lee JK, Choi IS, Song CE, Namgoong SK, Lee S. Journal of the American Chemical Society. 2004;**126**:480-481

[2] Chi YS, Lee JK, Lee SG, Choi IS. Langmuir. 2004;**20**:3024-3027

[3] Zhao Y, Li M, Lu Q. Langmuir. 2008;**24**:3937-3943

[4] Osicka J, Ilcikova M, Popelka A, Filip J, Bertok T, Tkac J, Kasak P. Langmuir. 2016; **32**:5491-5499

[5] Zhang Y, Shen Y, Yuan J, Han D, Wang Z, Zhang Q, Niu L. Angewandte Chemie International Edition. 2006;**45**:5867-5870

[6] Park MJ, Lee JK, Lee BS, Lee YW, Choi IS, Lee SG. Chemistry of Materials. 2006;**18**:1546-1551

[7] Dobbelin M, Marcilla R, Tollan C, Pomposo JA, Sarasua JR, Mecerreyes D. Journal of Materials Chemistry. 2008;**18**:5354-5358

[8] Shen Y, Zhang Y, Zhang Q, Niu L, You T, Ivaska A. Chemical Communications. 2005: 4193-4195

[9] He X, Yang W, Pei X. Macromolecules. 2008;**41**:4615-4621

[10] Law G, Watson PP. Langmuir. 2001;**17**:6138-6141

[11] Carvalho PJ, Freire MG, Marrucho IM, Queimada AJ, Coutinho JAP. Journal of Chemical and Engineering Data. 2008;**53**:1346-1350

[12] Azzaroni O, Brown AA, Huck WTS. Advanced Materials. 2007;**19**:151-154

[13] Wang L, Lin Y, Peng B, Su Z. Chemical Communications. 2008:5972-5974

[14] Azzaroni O, Moya S, Farhan T, Brown AA, Huck WTS. Macromolecules. 2005;**38**:10192-10199

[15] Zhou F, HY H, Yu B, Osborne VL, Huck WTS, Liu WM. Analytical Chemistry. 2007; **79**:176-182

[16] Lim HS, Lee SG, Lee DH, Lee DY, Lee S, Cho K. Advanced Materials. 2008;**20**:4438-4441

[17] Jiang C, Wang Q, Wang T. New Journal of Chemistry. 2013;**37**:810-814

[18] Jiang C, Wang Q, Wang T. New Journal of Chemistry. 2012;**36**:1641-1645

[19] Hua Z, Yang J, Wang T, Liu G, Zhang G. Langmuir. 2013;**29**:10307-10312

[20] Lee CH, Kang SK, Lim JA, Kwark YJ, Lim HS, Kim J, Cho JH. Journal of Materials Chemistry. 2012;**22**:14656-14660

[21] Wang L, Peng B, Su Z. Langmuir. 2010;**26**:12203-12208

[22] Zhang G, Zhang X, Huang Y, Su Z. ACS Applied Materials and Interfaces. 2013;**5**:6400-6403

[23] Zhang G, Zhang X, Li M, Su Z. ACS Applied Materials and Interfaces. 2014;**6**:1729-1733

[24] Yang F, Dong Y, Guo Z. Colloids and surfaces, A. 2014;**463**:101-109

[25] Ali N, Zhang B, Zhang H, Zaman W, Li X. Colloids and surfaces, A. 2015;**472**:38-49

[26] Zhang J, Li Y, Bao M, Yang X, Wang Z. Environmental Science and Technology. 2016;**50**:8809-8816

[27] Calcagnile P, Fragouli D, Bayer IS, Anyfantis GC, Martiradonna L, Cozzoli PD, Cingolani R, Athanassiou A. ACS Nano. 2012;**6**:5413-5419

[28] Wu L, Li L, Li B, Zhang J, Wang A. ACS Applied Materials and Interfaces. 2015;**7**:4936-4946

[29] Wu J, Wang N, Zhao Y, Jiang L. Nanoscale. 2015;**7**:2625-2632

[30] Zhang J, Feng H, Zao W, Zhao Y, Zhang H, Liu Y. RSC Advances. 2015;**5**:47892-47899

[31] Li L, Zhang J. Advanced Materials Interfaces. 2016;**3**:1600517/1-1600517/7

[32] Du R, Zhao Q, Li P, Ren H, Gao X, Zhang J. ACS Applied Materials and Interfaces. 2016;**8**:1025-1032

[33] Su C, Yang H, Song S, Lu B, Chen R. Chemical Engineering Journal. 2017;**309**:3636-3373

[34] Peng H, Wang H, Wu J, Meng G, Wang Y, Shi Y, Liu Z, Guo X. Industrial and Engineering Chemistry Research. 2016;**55**:832-838

[35] Cheng M, Ju G, Jiang C, Zhang Y, Shi F. Journal of Materials Chemistry A. 2013; **1**:13411-13416

[36] Kim JH, Kang SM, Lee BJ, Ko H, Bae WG, Suh KY, Kwak MK, Jeong HE. Scientific Reports. 2015;**5**:17843

[37] Cheng Z, Feng L, Jiang L. Advanced Materials. 2008;**18**:3219-3225

[38] Timonen JVI, Latikka M, Leibler L, Ras RHA, Ikkala O. Science. 2013;**341**:253-257

[39] Hong X, Gao X, Jiang L. Journal of the American Chemical Society. 2007;**129**:1478-1479

[40] Zhang JL, Li J, Han YC. Macromolecular Rapid Communications. 2004;**25**:1105-1108

[41] Zhang JL, XY L, Huang WH, Han YC. Macromolecular Rapid Communications. 2005; **26**:477-480

[42] Wu D, SZ W, Chen QD, Zhang YL, Yao J, Yao X, Niu LG, Wang JN, Jiang L, Sun HB. Advanced Materials. 2011;**23**:545-549

[43] Wu SZ, Wang JN, Niu LG, Yao J, Wu D, Li AW. Applied Physics Letters. 2011;**98**: 081902/1-081902/3

[44] Vasileiou T, Gerber J, Prautzsch J, Schutzius TM, Poulikakos D. Proceedings of the National Academy of Sciences U.S.A. 2016;**98**:081902/1-081902/3

[45] Liu Y, Andrew M, Li J, Yeomans JM, Wang Z. Nature Communications. 2015;**6** 10034

[46] Goel P, Kumar S, Sarkar J, Singh JP. ASC Applied MaterialsInterfaces. 2015;**7**:8419-8426

[47] Lin PC, Yang S. Soft Matter. 2009;**5**:1011-1018

[48] Liu Y, Liu Y, Hu H, Liu Z, Pei X, Yu B, Yan P, Zhou F. Journal of Physical Chemistry. C. 2015;**119**:7109-7114

[49] Zhu X, Zhang Z, Wang K, Yang J, Xu X, Men X, Zhou X. New Journal of Chemistry. 2012;**36**:1280-1284

[50] Zhu X, Zhang Z, Men X, Yang J, Xu X, Zhou X. Applied Surface Science. 2011;**257**:3753-3757

[51] Liu J, Chen F, Zheng H, Liu S, Sun J, Huang S, Song J, Jin Z, Liu X. RSC Advances. 2016; **6**:79437-79447

[52] Wu J, Bai HJ, Zhang XB, JJ X, Chen HY. Langmuir. 2010;**26**:1191-1198

[53] Yang Y, Li H, Cheng S, Zou G, Wang C, Lin Q. Chemical Communications. 2014;**50**: 2900-2903

[54] Pinchasik BE, Wang H, Möhwald H, Asanuma H. Advanced Materials Interfaces. 2016;**3**:1600722/1-1600722/6

[55] Feng N, Zhao H, Zhan J, Tian D, Li H. Organic Letters. 2012;**14**:1958-1961

[56] Zhang GF, Zhan JY, Li HB. Organic Letters. 2011;**13**:3392-3395

[57] Xu L, Liu N, Cao Y, Lu F, Chen Y, Zhang X, Feng L, Wei Y. ACS Applied Materials and Interfaces. 2014;**6**:13324-13329

[58] Rodriguez-Hermida S, Tsang MY, Vignatti C, Stylianou KC, Guillerm V, Perez-Carvajal J, Teixidor F, Vinas C, Choquesillo-Lazarte D, Verdugo-Escamilla C, Peral I, Juanhuix J, Verdaguer A, Imaz I, Maspoch D, Planas JG. Angewandte Chemie International Edition. 2016;**55**:1-6

[59] Rao KV, Mohapatra S, Maji TK, George SJ. Chemistry - A European Journal. 2012;**18**: 4505-4509

[60] Qing G, Wang X, Fuchs H, Sun T. Journal of American Chemical Society. 2009;**131**:8370-8371

[61] Qing G, Wang X, Jiang L, Fuchs H, Sun T. Soft Matter. 2009;**5**:2759-2765

[62] Boyes SG, Brittain WJ, Wang X, Cheng SZD. Macromolecules. 2002;**35**:4960-4967

[63] Jennings GK, Brantley EL. Advanced Materials. 2004;**16**:1983-1994

[64] Zhao B, Brittain WJ. Macromolecules. 2000;**33**:8813-8820

[65] Tan H, Sun TL, Li JH, Guo M, Xie XY, Zhong YP, Fu Q, Jiang L. Macromolecular Rapid Communications. 2005;**26**:1418-1422

[66] Julthongpiput D, Lin YH, Teng J, Zubarev ER, Tsukruk VV. Journal of the American Chemical Society. 2003;**125**:912-915

[67] Julthongpiput D, Lin Y, Teng J, Zubarev ER, Tsukruk VV. Langmuir. 2003;**19**:7832-7836

[68] Yang J, Zhang Z, Men X, Xu X, Zhu X. Journal of Colloid and Interface Science. 2010; **346**:241-247

[69] Minko S, Muller M, Motornov M, Nitschke M, Grundke K, Stamm M. Journal of the American Chemical Society. 2003;**125**:3896-3900

[70] Sidorenko A, Minko S, Schenk-Meuser K, Duschner H, Stamm M. Langmuir. 1999;**15**: 8349-8355

[71] Shen L, Fu J, Fu K, Picart C, Ji J. Langmuir. 2010;**26**:16634-16637

[72] Li Y, Li X, Guo W, Wu M, Sun J. Science China Chemistry. 2016;**59**:1568-1573

[73] Sidorenko A, Krupenkin T, Aizenberg J. Journal of Materials Chemistry. 2008;**18**: 38418-33846

[74] Heng L, Dong Y, Zhai J, Tang B, Jiang L. Langmuir. 2008;**24**:2157-2161

[75] Tokudome Y, Okada K, Nakahira A, Takahashi M. Journal of Materials Chemistry A. 2014;**2**:58-61

[76] Lian Z, Xu J, Wang Z, Weng Z, Xu Z, Yu H. Applied Surface Science. 2016;**390**:244-247

[77] Lv LB, Cui TL, Zhang B, Wang HH, Li XH, Chen JS. Angewandte Chemistry International Edition. 2015;**54**:15165-15169

[78] Liu N, Cao Y, Lin X, Chen Y, Feng L, Wei Y. ACS Applied Materials and Interfaces. 2014; **6**:12821-12826

[79] Basu BJ, Manasa J. Applied Physics A. 2011;**103**:343-348

[80] Zhu W, Zhai J, Sun Z, Jiang L. Journal of Physical Chemical C. 2008;**112**:8338-8342

[81] Wang J, Guo J, Si P, Cai W, Wang Y, Wu G. RSC Advances. 2016;**6**:4329-4334

[82] Si Y, Yang F, Guo Z. Journal of Colloid and Interface Science. 2016;**484**:173-182

[83] Che H, Huo M, Peng L, Fang T, Liu N, Feng L, Wei Y, Yuan J. Angewandte Chemistry, International Edition. 2015;**54**:8934-8938

[84] Zhang Y, Dong J, Sun H, Yu B, Zhu Z, Zhang J, Wang A. ACS Applied Materials and Interfaces. 2016;**8**:27346-27353

[85] Seo J, Lee JS, Lee K, Kim D, Yang K, Shin S, Mahata C, Jung HB, Lee W, Cho SW, Lee T. Advanced Materials. 2014;**26**:7043-7050

[86] Yadav K, Mehta BR, Bhattacharya S, Singh JP. Scientific Reports. 2016;**6**:35073

[87] Godeau G, Darmanin T, Guittard F. Reactive and Functional Polymers. 2015;**96**:44-49

[88] Taleb S, Noyer E, Godeau G, Darmanin T, Guittard F. Chemphyschem. 2016;**17**:305-309

[89] Godeau G, Darmanin T, Guittard F. Journal of Applied Polymer Science. 2016;**133** 43130

[90] Cheng Z, Lai H, Du M, Zhu S, Zhang N, Sun K. Soft Matter. 2012;**8**:9635-9641

[91] Xia F, Feng L, Wang S, Sun T, Song W, Jiang W, Jiang L. Advanced Materials. 2006;**18**:432-436

[92] Motornov M, Sheparovych R, Lupitskyy R, MacWilliams E, Minko S. Advanced Materials. 2008;**20**:200-205

[93] Motornov M, Sheparovych R, Lupitskyy R, MacWilliams E, Minko S. Journal of Colloid and Interface Science. 2007;**310**:481-488

[94] JD W, Zhang C, Jiang DJ, Zhao SF, Jiang YL, Cai GQ, Wang JP. RSC Advances. 2016; **6**:24076-24082

[95] Li T, Shen J, Zhang Z, Wang S, Wei D. RSC Advances. 2016;**6**:40656-60663

[96] Guo Y, Xia F, Xu L, Li J, Yang W, Jiang L. Langmuir. 2010;**26**:1024-1208

[97] Rodriguez-Hernandez J, Munoz-Bonilla A, Bousquet A, Ibarboure E, Papon E. Langmuir. 2010;**26**:18617-18620

[98] Tan L, Cao L, Yang M, Wang G, Sun D. Polymer. 2011;**52**:4770-4776

[99] Zhu Y, Feng L, Xia F, Zhai J, Wan M, Jiang L. Macromolecular Rapid Communications. 2007;**28**:1135-1141

[100] Darmanin T, Guittard F. Chemphyschem. 2013;**14**:2529-2533

[101] Doebbelin M, Tena-Zaera R, Marcilla R, Iturri J, Moya S, Pomposo JA, Mecerreyes D. Advanced Functional Materials. 2009;**19**:3326-3333

[102] Doebbelin M, Pozo-Gonzalo C, Marcilla R, Blanco R, Segura JL, Pomposo JA, Mecerreyes D. Journal of Polymer Science, Part A: Polymer Chemistry. 2009;**47**:3010-3021

[103] Doebbelin M, Marcilla R, Tollan C, Pomposo JA, Sarasua JR, Mecerreyes D. Journal of Materials Chemistry. 2008;**18**:5354-5358

[104] Taleb S, Darmanin T, Guittard F. ACS Applied Materials and Interfaces. 2014;**6**:7953-7960

[105] Taleb S, Darmanin T, Guittard F. RSC Advances. 2014;**4**:3550-3555

[106] Taleb S, Darmanin T, Guittard F. Materials Today Communications. 2016;**6**:1-8

[107] Li HL, Xin BW, Feng L, Hao JC. Science China Chemistry. 2014;**57**:1002-1009

[108] Peng Y, He Y, Yang S, Ben S, Cao M, Li K, Liu K, Jiang L. Advanced Functional Materials. 2015;**25**:5967-5971

[109] Grigoryev A, Tokarev I, Kornev KG, Luzinov I, Minko S. Journal of the American Chemical Society. 2012;**134**:12916-12919

[110] Sun W, Zhou S, You B, Wu L. Journal of Materials Chemistry A. 2013;**1**:3146-3154

[111] Xia F, Ge H, Hou Y, Sun T, Chen L, Zhang G, Jiang L. Advanced Materials. 2007;**19**:2520-2524